POCKET ATLAS
OF
ANATOMY

POCKET ATLAS

OF

ANATOMY

BY
VICTOR PAUCHET AND S. DUPRET

THIRD EDITION
345 PLATES

OXFORD UNIVERSITY PRESS
NEW YORK MELBOURNE

Oxford University Press, Walton Street, Oxford OX2 6DP

London Glasgow New York Toronto
Delhi Bombay Calcutta Madras Karachi
Kuala Lumpur Singapore Hong Kong Tokyo
Nairobi Dar es Salaam Cape Town
Melbourne Auckland
and associated companies in
Beirut Berlin Ibadan Mexico City Nicosia

OXFORD is a trade mark of Oxford University Press

© *Oxford University Press 1928*
Third edition 1937
Eleventh impression 1983

ISBN 0 19 263131 4

Printed in Hong Kong

PREFACE TO THE THIRD EDITION

THE names used in the third edition are taken from the nomenclature adopted by the Anatomical Society at Birmingham in 1933 ; but where they differ markedly from the Basle Nomina Anatomica, the B.N.A. are retained in square brackets.

PREFACE TO THE SECOND ENGLISH EDITION

IN the new edition twenty-eight new plates have been added, and some alterations and corrections have been made in the old plates and an index and alphabetical list of plates have been supplied.

PREFACE TO THE FIRST EDITION

I USED to teach anatomy and operative surgery in the Medical School at Amiens, where my lectures were always given, scalpel in hand. There was no lack of subjects. My notes would have been allowed to perish had I not met with the anatomical draughtsman S. Dupret, an artist whose extraordinary powers of draughtsmanship, keen intelligence, devotion to work, and anatomical skill made the preparation of this book possible.

I submitted my project to my friend Gaston Doin, who, with skilled craftsmen to help, took up my idea and realised it without delay.

We have founded great hopes on this offspring of us three, for it carries in it the germ of success—convenience. We would like to see it in the hands of all students in the dissecting-room and in the wards : at the dissecting-table or by the bedside it will recall the facts of anatomy at once and without trouble—there is no text and no legends. We would like it to find place in the pockets of candidates for all examinations. In the omnibus or on the seats in the Luxembourg Gardens they can here revise, rapidly, the names and relations of the various structures. We would like it to find its way into the hospital, and into the surgeon's room, who, before an unusual operation, could, in five minutes, refresh his memory of the relations of the structures in the area in which he proposes to operate.

The book no doubt contains omissions and defects—these we will remedy as they come to light, trusting that the reader will bring them directly under our notice.

VICTOR PAUCHET.

ALPHABETICAL LIST OF PLATES

ATLAS

PLATE 1.—FRONT VIEW OF HUMAN SKELETON WITH SKIN CONTOUR

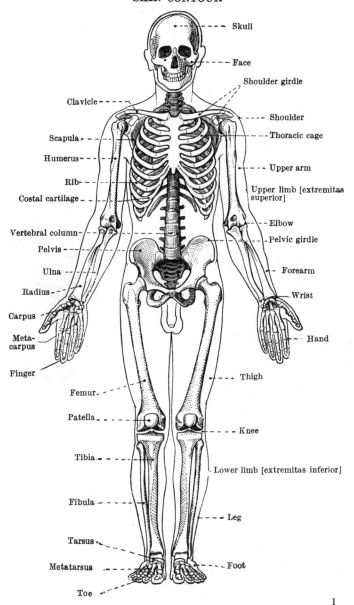

Skull

Face

Shoulder girdle

Clavicle

Shoulder

Scapula

Thoracic cage

Humerus

Upper arm

Rib

Upper limb [extremitas superior]

Costal cartilage

Vertebral column

Elbow

Pelvis

Pelvic girdle

Ulna

Forearm

Radius

Wrist

Carpus

Meta-carpus

Hand

Finger

Thigh

Femur

Patella

Knee

Tibia

Lower limb [extremitas inferior]

Fibula

Leg

Tarsus

Metatarsus

Foot

Toe

PLATE 2.—FRONTAL BONE

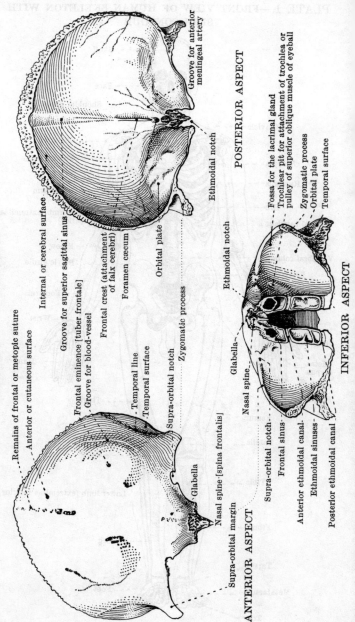

ANTERIOR ASPECT

- Remains of frontal or metopic suture
- Anterior or cutaneous surface
- Frontal eminence [tuber frontale]
- Groove for blood-vessel
- Temporal line
- Temporal surface
- Supra-orbital notch
- Zygomatic process
- Glabella
- Nasal spine [spina frontalis]
- Supra-orbital margin

POSTERIOR ASPECT

- Internal or cerebral surface
- Groove for superior sagittal sinus
- Frontal crest (attachment of falx cerebri)
- Foramen caecum
- Orbital plate
- Ethmoidal notch
- Groove for anterior meningeal artery

INFERIOR ASPECT

- Fossa for the lacrimal gland
- Trochlear pit for attachment of trochlea or pulley of superior oblique muscle of eyeball
- Zygomatic process
- Orbital plate
- Temporal surface
- Ethmoidal notch
- Glabella
- Nasal spine
- Supra-orbital notch
- Frontal sinus
- Anterior ethmoidal canal
- Ethmoidal sinuses
- Posterior ethmoidal canal

PLATE 3.—ETHMOID BONE

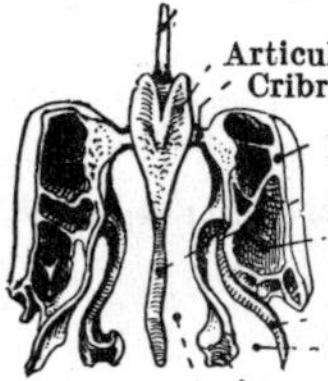

SUPERIOR ASPECT

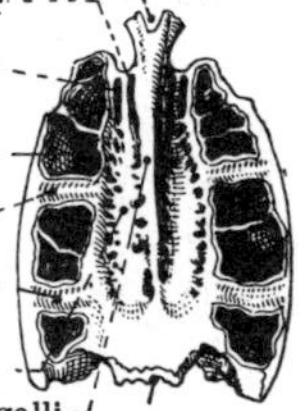

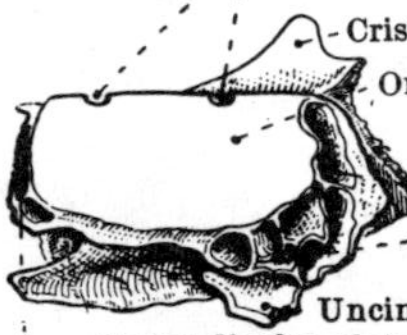

Notch completing foramen caecum
Groove for process of dura mater
Foramen for anterior ethmoidal artery and nerve
Infundibulum (continuous with frontal sinus)
Anterior and posterior ethmoidal grooves (for vessels and nerve)
Cribriform plate with foramina for olfactory nerves
Crista galli
Posterior border

POSTERIOR ASPECT

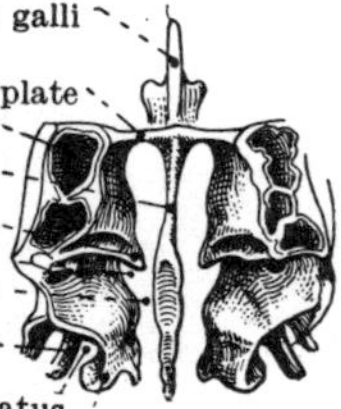

Crista galli
Cribriform plate
Posterior ethmoidal sinuses
Perpendicular plate
Superior concha of the nose
Superior meatus
Left nasal cavity
Uncinate process
Middle meatus
Middle concha of the nose

ANTERIOR ASPECT

Crista galli
Articular surface for frontal bone
Cribriform plate
Ethmoidal labyrinth
Perpendicular plate
Anterior ethmoidal sinuses
Uncinate process
Middle meatus
Left nasal cavity

RIGHT LATERAL ASPECT

Anterior and posterior ethmoidal canals
Crista galli
Orbital plate [lamina papyracea]
Perpendicular plate
Anterior ethmoidal sinuses
Middle concha (lateral surface) and middle meatus of nose
Uncinate process
Perpendicular plate
Posterior ethmoidal sinuses

PLATE 4.—SPHENOID BONE

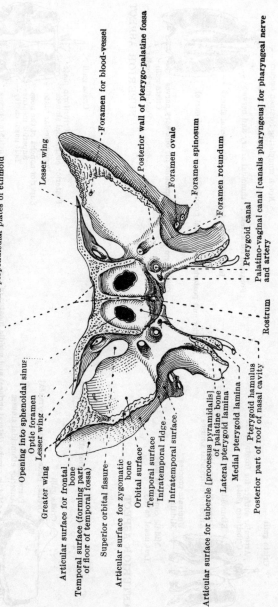

Articular surfaces for cribriform and perpendicular plates of ethmoid

Opening into sphenoidal sinus:
Optic foramen
Lesser wing

Articular surface for frontal bone
Temporal surface (forming part of floor of temporal fossa)

Greater wing
Lesser wing

Articular surface for zygomatic bone
Orbital surface
Superior orbital fissure
Temporal surface
Infratemporal ridge
Infratemporal surface

Articular surface for tubercle [processus pyramidalis] of palatine bone
Lateral pterygoid lamina
Medial pterygoid lamina
Pterygoid hamulus
Posterior part of roof of nasal cavity

Foramen for blood-vessel

Posterior wall of pterygo-palatine fossa
Foramen ovale
Foramen spinosum
Foramen rotundum

Pterygoid canal
Palatino-vaginal canal [canalis pharyngeus] for pharyngeal nerve and artery

Rostrum

ANTERIOR ASPECT

PLATE 5.—SPHENOID BONE

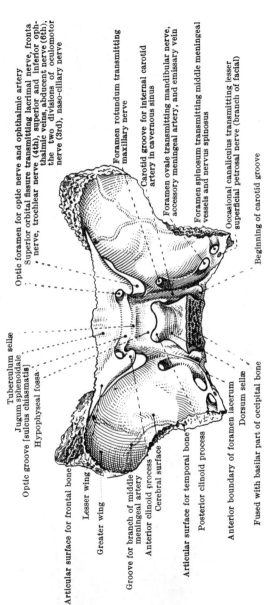

Tuberculum sellæ
Optic groove [sulcus chiasmatis]
Jugum sphenoidale
Hypophyseal fossa

Optic foramen for optic nerve and ophthalmic artery
Superior orbital fissure transmitting lacrimal nerve, frontal nerve, trochlear nerve (4th), superior and inferior ophthalmic veins, abducent nerve (6th), the two divisions of oculomotor nerve (3rd), naso-ciliary nerve

Foramen rotundum transmitting maxillary nerve

Carotid groove for internal carotid artery in cavernous sinus

Foramen ovale transmitting mandibular nerve, accessory meningeal artery, and emissary vein

Foramen spinosum transmitting middle meningeal vessels and nervus spinosus

Occasional canaliculus transmitting lesser superficial petrosal nerve (branch of facial)

Beginning of carotid groove

Articular surface for frontal bone
Lesser wing
Greater wing
Groove for branch of middle meningeal artery
Anterior clinoid process
Cerebral surface
Articular surface for temporal bone
Posterior clinoid process

Anterior boundary of foramen lacerum
Dorsum sellæ

Fused with basilar part of occipital bone

SUPERIOR ASPECT

PLATE 6.—PARIETAL BONE

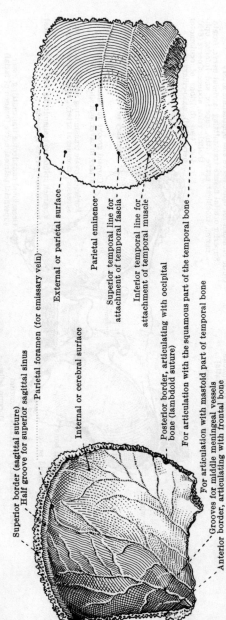

Superior border (sagittal suture)
Half groove for superior sagittal sinus
Parietal foramen (for emissary vein)
External or parietal surface
Internal or cerebral surface
Parietal eminence
Superior temporal line for attachment of temporal fascia
Inferior temporal line for attachment of temporal muscle
Posterior border, articulating with occipital bone (lambdoid suture)
For articulation with the squamous part of the temporal bone
For articulation with mastoid part of temporal bone
Grooves for middle meningeal vessels
Anterior border, articulating with frontal bone

INTERNAL OR CEREBRAL SURFACE

EXTERNAL OR PARIETAL SURFACE

PLATE 7.—OCCIPITAL BONE

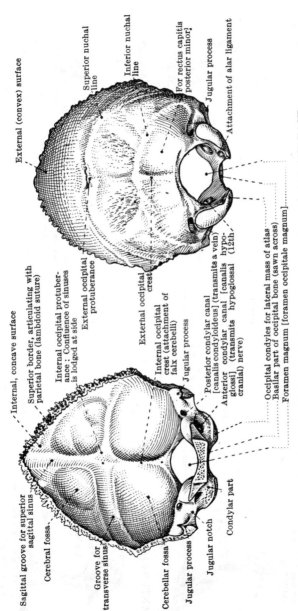

INTERNAL OR CEREBRAL SURFACE

EXTERNAL SURFACE

Internal, concave surface

Superior border, articulating with parietal bone (lambdoid suture)

Internal occipital protuberance : Confluence of sinuses is lodged at side

External occipital protuberance

External occipital crest

Internal occipital crest (attachment of falx cerebelli)

Jugular process

Posterior condylar canal [canalis condyloideus] (transmits a vein)

Anterior condylar canal [canalis hypoglossi] (transmits hypoglossal (12th) cranial) nerve)

Occipital condyles for lateral mass of atlas

Basilar part of occipital bone (sawn across)

Foramen magnum [foramen occipitale magnum]

Sagittal groove for superior sagittal sinus

Cerebral fossa

Groove for transverse sinus

Cerebellar fossa

Jugular process

Jugular notch

Condylar part

External (convex) surface

Superior nuchal line

Inferior nuchal line

For rectus capitis posterior minor

Jugular process

Attachment of alar ligament

PLATE 8.—PALATINE BONE.

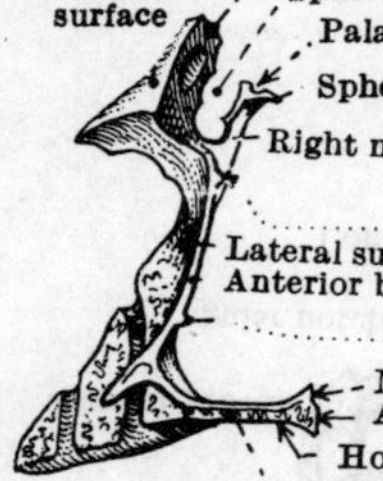

Articular surfaces for sphenoid bone
Spheno-palatine notch
Articular surface for ethmoid bone
Opening of one of the posterior ethmoidal sinuses
Posterior part of superior meatus
Middle meatus
Sphenoidal process
Inferior meatus
Tubercle [processus pyramidalis]

MEDIAL ASPECT

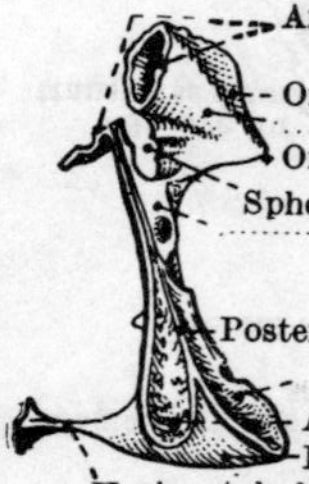

Anterior border
Orbital surface
Palatino-vaginal canal (c. pharyngeus) (half)
Posterior border
Articular surface for maxilla
Medial wall of pterygo-palatine fossa
Palatino-vaginal canal [c. pharyngeus] (half)
Medial wall of pterygo-palatine fossa
Surface towards and in part closing the opening of maxillary sinus
Articular surface for maxilla
Articular surface for lateral pterygoid plate
Greater palatine canal (c. pterygo-palatinus)
completed by articulation with maxilla

LATERAL ASPECT

Orbital
process
Orbital
surface
Spheno-palatine notch
Palatino-vaginal canal (c. pharyngeus) (half)
Sphenoidal process
Anterior border
Right nasal cavity
Lateral surface articulating with maxilla
Ethmoidal crest for articulation with maxilla
Conchal crest for articulation with posterior end of inferior concha
Nasal crest for posterior part of inferior border of vomer
Articular surface for horizontal plate of left palatine bone
Horizontal plate [pars horizontalis]
Articular surface for palatine process of maxilla

ANTERIOR ASPECT

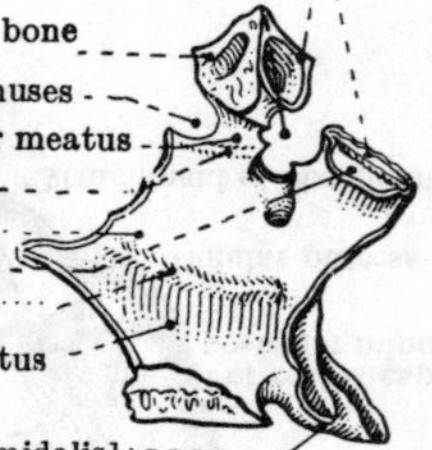

Articular surfaces for sphenoid bone
Orbital surface
Orbital process
Spheno-palatine notch
Posterior border
Articular surface for medial pterygoid plate
Pterygoid fossa
Horizontal plate [pars horizontalis]

POSTERIOR ASPECT

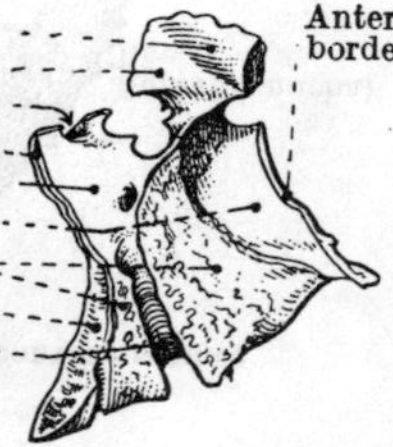

PLATE 9.—TEMPORAL BONE

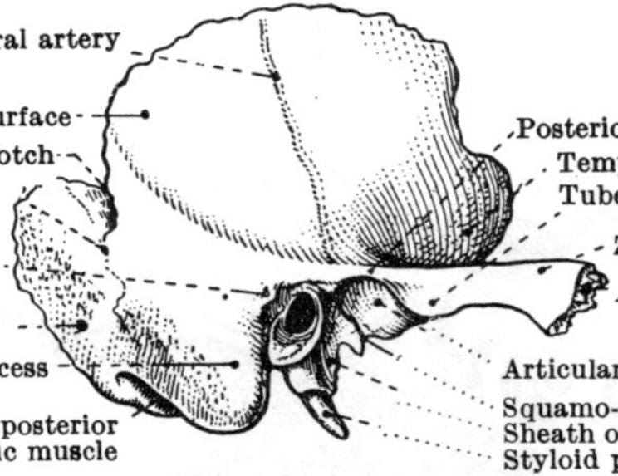

Groove for middle temporal artery

Squamous part : external or temporal surface
Parietal notch
Remains of squamo-mastoid suture

Supra-meatal spine

Mastoid foramen transmitting an emissary vein
and a small branch of the occipital artery
Mastoid process

Mastoid notch : origin of posterior
belly of digastric muscle

Posterior root of zygoma
Temporal fossa
Tubercle of root of zygoma

Zygomatic process or zygoma

Articular surface for zygomatic bone

Articular fossa [f. mandibularis] for head of mandible
Squamo-tympanic fissure [f. petrotympanica]
Sheath of styloid process
Styloid process

LATERAL ASPECT

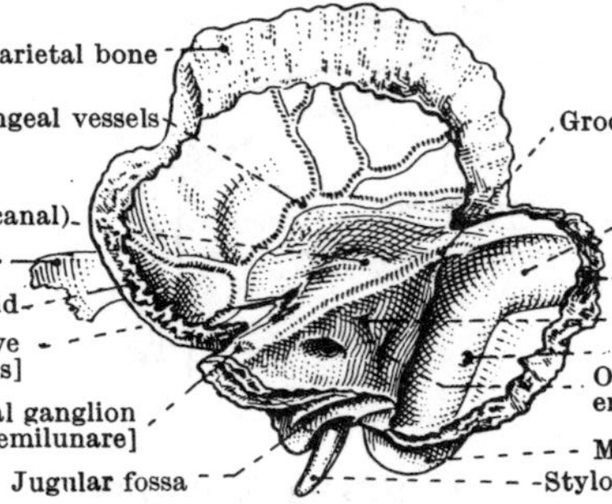

Groove for superior petrosal sinus

Groove for sigmoid sinus
Articular surface for occipital bone
Fossa subarcuata
Mastoid foramen
Opening of the aqueductus vestibuli (for ductus
endolymphaticus)
Mastoid process
Styloid process

Articular surface for parietal bone

Grooves for branches of the middle meningeal vessels

Arcuate eminence (made by sup. semicircular canal)
Zygomatic process or zygoma
Articular surface for greater wing of sphenoid
Slit for greater superficial petrosal nerve
[hiatus canalis facialis]
Impression for trigeminal ganglion
[g. semilunare]
Jugular fossa

MEDIAL ASPECT

PLATE 10.—VERTICAL SECTION THROUGH THE AUDITORY APPARATUS

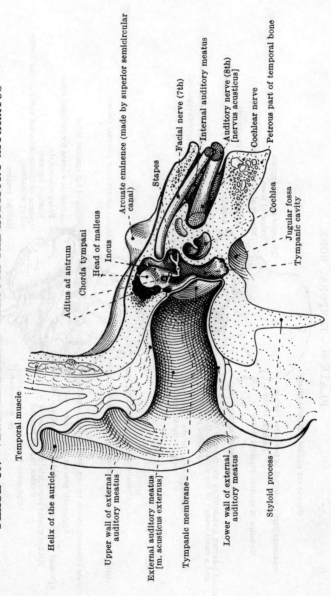

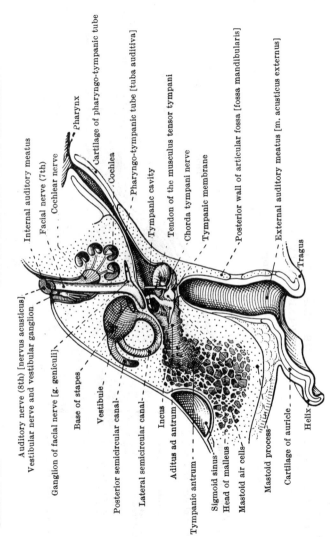

PLATE 11.—HORIZONTAL SECTION THROUGH THE AUDITORY APPARATUS

Auditory nerve (8th) [nervus acusticus]
Vestibular nerve and vestibular ganglion
Internal auditory meatus
Facial nerve (7th)
Cochlear nerve
Pharynx
Cartilage of pharyngo-tympanic tube
Cochlea
Pharyngo-tympanic tube [tuba auditiva]
Tympanic cavity
Tendon of the musculus tensor tympani
Chorda tympani nerve
Tympanic membrane
Posterior wall of articular fossa [fossa mandibularis]
External auditory meatus [m. acusticus externus]
Tragus
Ganglion of facial nerve [g. geniculi]
Base of stapes
Vestibule
Posterior semicircular canal
Lateral semicircular canal
Incus
Aditus ad antrum
Tympanic antrum
Sigmoid sinus
Head of malleus
Mastoid air cells
Mastoid process
Cartilage of auricle
Helix

PLATE 12.—SECTION THROUGH TEMPORAL BONE, SHOWING MEDIAL WALL OF TYMPANIC CAVITY, ETC.

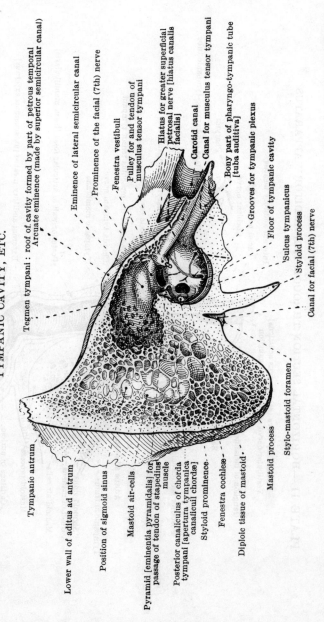

Tegmen tympani : roof of cavity formed by part of petrous temporal
Arcuate eminence (made by superior semicircular canal)

Eminence of lateral semicircular canal

Prominence of the facial (7th) nerve

Fenestra vestibuli

Pulley for and tendon of
musculus tensor tympani

Hiatus for greater superficial
petrosal nerve [hiatus canalis
facialis]

Carotid canal

Canal for musculus tensor tympani

Bony part of pharyngo-tympanic tube
[tuba auditiva]

Grooves for tympanic plexus

Floor of tympanic cavity

Sulcus tympanicus

Styloid process

Canal for facial (7th) nerve

Tympanic antrum

Lower wall of aditus ad antrum

Position of sigmoid sinus

Mastoid air-cells

Pyramid [eminentia pyramidalis] for
passage of tendon of stapedius
muscle

Posterior canaliculus of chorda
tympani [apertura tympanica
canaliculi chordae]

Styloid prominence

Fenestra cochleae

Diploic tissue of mastoid

Mastoid process

Stylo-mastoid foramen

PLATE 13

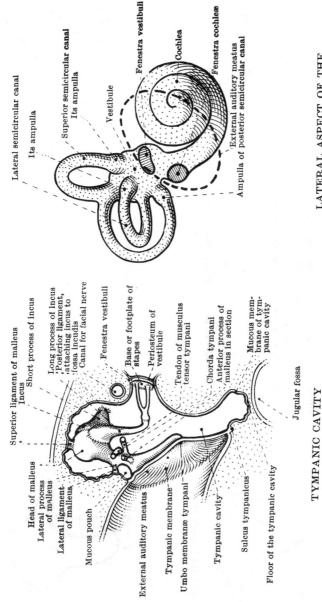

Superior ligament of malleus
Incus
Short process of incus

Long process of incus
Posterior ligament, attaching incus to fossa incudis
Canal for facial nerve

Fenestra vestibuli

Base or footplate of stapes
Periosteum of vestibule

Tendon of musculus tensor tympani

Chorda tympani
Anterior process of malleus in section

Mucous membrane of tympanic cavity

Head of malleus
Lateral process of malleus
Lateral ligament of malleus

Mucous pouch

External auditory meatus

Tympanic membrane

Umbo membranae tympani

Tympanic cavity

Sulcus tympanicus

Floor of the tympanic cavity

Jugular fossa

TYMPANIC CAVITY

Lateral semicircular canal
Its ampulla

Superior semicircular canal
Its ampulla

Vestibule

Fenestra vestibuli

Cochlea

Fenestra cochleae

External auditory meatus

Ampulla of posterior semicircular canal

**LATERAL ASPECT OF THE
MEMBRANOUS LABYRINTH**

PLATE 14.—ZYGOMATIC BONE

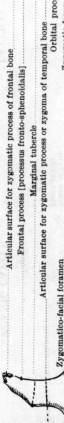

Articular surface for zygomatic process of frontal bone
Frontal process [processus fronto-sphenoidalis]
Marginal tubercle
Articular surface for zygomatic process or zygoma of temporal bone
Orbital process
Zygomatic foramen

Articular surface for maxilla

Zygomatico-temporal foramen transmitting zygomatico-temporal nerve

Zygomatico-facial foramen

MEDIAL ASPECT

LATERAL ASPECT

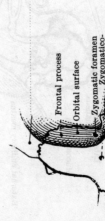

Frontal process
Temporal surface

Zygomatico-temporal foramen transmitting zygomatico-temporal nerve

Zygomatic process of temporal

Maxilla

Zygomatic process of frontal bone

POSTERIOR ASPECT

Frontal process
Orbital surface
Zygomatic foramen
Zygomatico-facial foramen

ANTERIOR ASPECT

PLATE 15.—MAXILLA

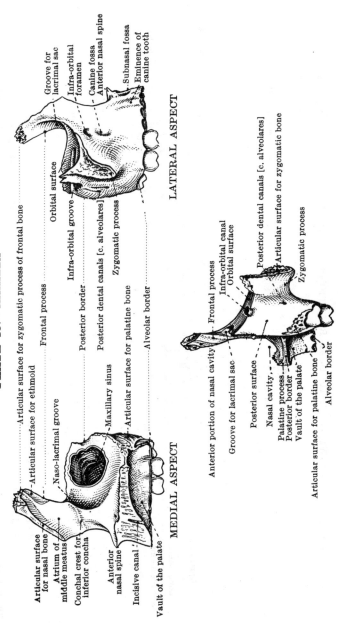

LATERAL ASPECT

Groove for lacrimal sac
Infra-orbital foramen
Canine fossa
Anterior nasal spine
Subnasal fossa
Eminence of canine tooth

Articular surface for zygomatic process of frontal bone
Frontal process
Orbital surface
Posterior border
Infra-orbital groove
Posterior dental canals [c. alveolares]
Zygomatic process

POSTERIOR ASPECT

Frontal process
Infra-orbital canal
Orbital surface
Posterior dental canals [c. alveolares]
Articular surface for zygomatic bone
Zygomatic process

Anterior portion of nasal cavity
Groove for lacrimal sac
Posterior surface
Nasal cavity
Palatine process
Posterior border
Vault of the palate
Articular surface for palatine bone
Alveolar border

MEDIAL ASPECT

Articular surface for ethmoid
Naso-lacrimal groove
Maxillary sinus
Articular surface for palatine bone
Alveolar border

Articular surface for nasal bone
Atrium of middle meatus
Conchal crest for inferior concha
Anterior nasal spine
Incisive canal
Vault of the palate

PLATE 16.—SHOWING RECIPROCAL RELATIONS OF UPPER AND LOWER TEETH

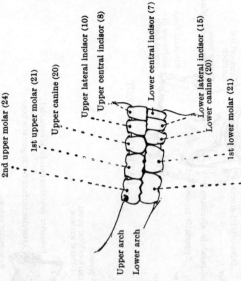

2nd upper molar (24)

1st upper molar (21)

Upper canine (20)

Upper lateral incisor (10)

Upper central incisor (8)

Upper central incisor (7)

Lower lateral incisor (15)

Lower canine (20)

1st lower molar (21)

2nd lower molar (24)

Upper arch

Lower arch

FIRST DENTITION
TEMPORARY OR MILK TEETH
[DENTES DECIDUI]

The numbers in brackets represent the age in months when the various teeth erupt.

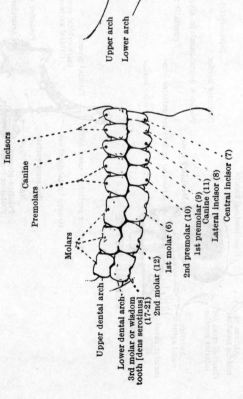

Incisors

Canine

Premolars

Molars

Upper dental arch

Lower dental arch

3rd molar or wisdom tooth [dens serotinus] (17-21)

2nd molar (12)

1st molar (6)

2nd premolar (10)

1st premolar (9)

Canine (11)

Lateral incisor (8)

Central incisor (7)

SECOND DENTITION
PERMANENT TEETH

The numbers in brackets indicate the year during or soon after which the teeth erupt; those of the upper jaw appear a little later.

PLATE 17.—PERMANENT TEETH

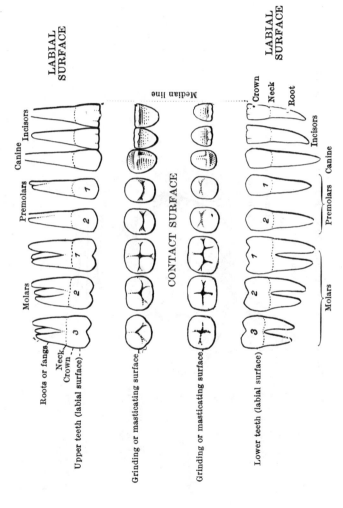

LABIAL SURFACE

Canine Incisors

Premolars

Molars

Roots or fangs
Neck
Crown (labial surface)

Upper teeth (labial surface)

Grinding or masticating surface

Median line

CONTACT SURFACE

Grinding or masticating surface

Crown
Neck
Root

Incisors

Canine

Premolars

Molars

Lower teeth (labial surface)

LABIAL SURFACE

2

PLATE 18.—BONY SKELETON OF RIGHT NASAL CAVITY

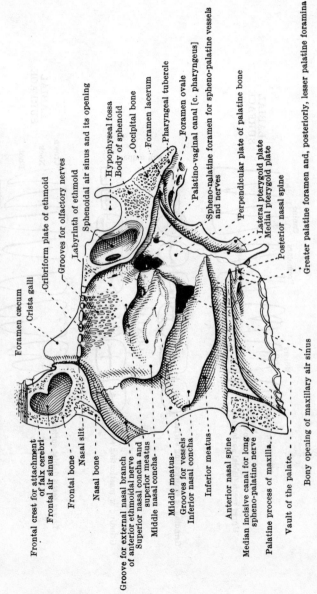

Frontal crest for attachment of falx cerebri
Frontal air sinus
Nasal slit
Frontal bone
Nasal bone
Groove for external nasal branch of anterior ethmoidal nerve
Superior nasal concha and superior meatus
Middle nasal concha
Middle meatus
Grooves for vessels
Inferior nasal concha
Inferior meatus
Anterior nasal spine
Median incisive canal for long spheno-palatine nerve
Palatine process of maxilla
Vault of the palate.
Bony opening of maxillary air sinus

Foramen caecum
Crista galli
Cribriform plate of ethmoid
Grooves for olfactory nerves
Labyrinth of ethmoid
Sphenoidal air sinus and its opening
Hypophyseal fossa
Body of sphenoid
Occipital bone
Foramen lacerum
Pharyngeal tubercle
Foramen ovale
Spheno-palatine foramen for spheno-palatine vessels and nerves
Palatino-vaginal canal [c. pharyngeus]
Perpendicular plate of palatine bone
Lateral pterygoid plate
Medial pterygoid plate
Posterior nasal spine
Greater palatine foramen and, posteriorly, lesser palatine foramina

PLATE 19.—RIGHT NASAL CAVITY WITH ITS MUCOUS MEMBRANE

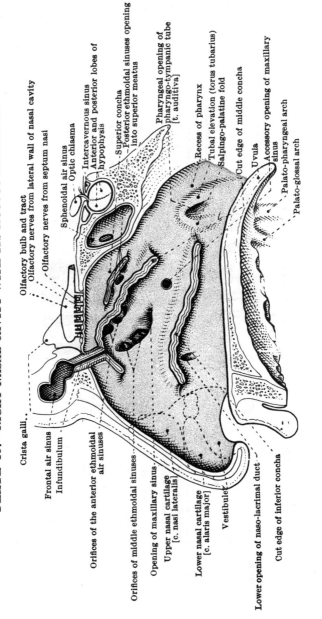

Crista galli

Frontal air sinus
Infundibulum

Orifices of the anterior ethmoidal air sinuses

Orifices of middle ethmoidal sinuses

Opening of maxillary sinus
Upper nasal cartilage [c. nasi lateralis]

Lower nasal cartilage [c. alaris major]
Vestibule

Lower opening of naso-lacrimal duct
Cut edge of inferior concha

Olfactory bulb and tract
Olfactory nerves from lateral wall of nasal cavity
Olfactory nerves from septum nasi

Sphenoidal air sinus
Optic chiasma
Intercavernous sinus
Anterior and posterior lobes of hypophysis
Superior concha
Posterior ethmoidal sinuses opening into superior meatus
Pharyngeal opening of pharyngo-tympanic tube [t. auditiva]
Recess of pharynx
Tubal elevation (torus tubarius)
Salpingo-palatine fold
Cut edge of middle concha
Uvula
Accessory opening of maxillary sinus
Palato-pharyngeal arch
Palato-glossal arch

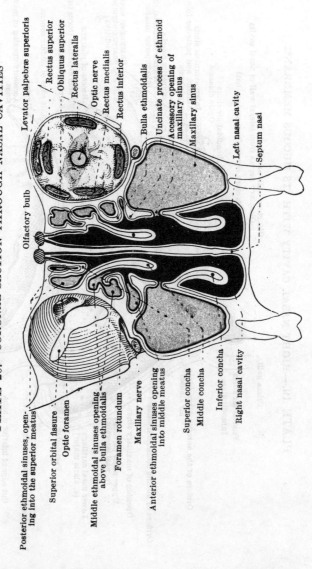

PLATE 20.—CORONAL SECTION THROUGH NASAL CAVITIES

Rectus superior
Levator palpebræ superioris
Obliquus superior
Rectus lateralis

Optic nerve
Rectus medialis
Rectus inferior

Olfactory bulb

Bulla ethmoidalis
Uncinate process of ethmoid
Accessory opening of maxillary sinus
Maxillary sinus

Left nasal cavity

Septum nasi

Posterior ethmoidal sinuses, opening into the superior meatus

Superior orbital fissure
Optic foramen

Middle ethmoidal sinuses opening above bulla ethmoidalis

Foramen rotundum

Maxillary nerve

Anterior ethmoidal sinuses opening into middle meatus

Superior concha
Middle concha

Inferior concha

Right nasal cavity

PLATE 21.—MANDIBLE

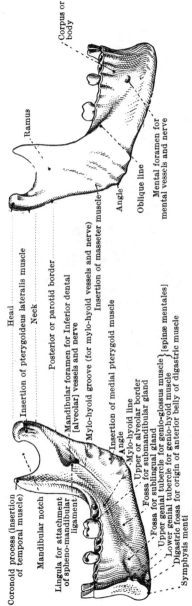

Coronoid process (insertion of temporal muscle)

Mandibular notch

Lingula for attachment of spheno-mandibular ligament

Head

Insertion of pterygoideus lateralis muscle

Neck

Posterior or parotid border

Mandibular foramen for Inferior dental [alveolar] vessels and nerve

Mylo-hyoid groove (for mylo-hyoid vessels and nerve)

Insertion of medial pterygoid muscle

Angle

Mylo-hyoid line

Upper or alveolar border

Fossa for sublingual gland

Fossa for submandibular gland

Upper genial tubercle for genio-glossus muscle] [spinae mentales]

Lower genial tubercle for genio-hyoid muscle

Digastric fossa for origin of anterior belly of digastric muscle

Symphysis menti

MEDIAL ASPECT

Ramus

Corpus or body

Angle

Oblique line

Mental foramen for Mental vessels and nerve

Insertion of masseter muscle

LATERAL ASPECT

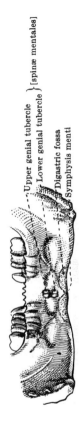

Upper genial tubercle ⎱ [spinae mentales]
Lower genial tubercle ⎰

Digastric fossa

Symphysis menti

BODY OF MANDIBLE—POSTERIOR ASPECT

PLATE 22.—FRONT OF SKULL.

Attachments of Muscles.   O. = Origin.   I. = Insertion.

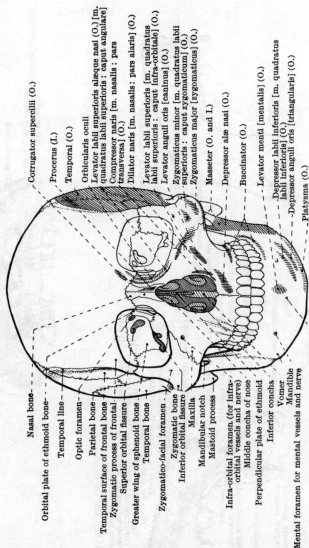

Corrugator supercilii (O.)
Procerus (I.)
Temporal (O.)
Orbicularis oculi
Levator labii superioris alaeque nasi (O.) [m. quadratus labii superioris : caput angulare]
Compressor naris [m. nasalis : pars transversa] (O.)
Dilator naris [m. nasalis : pars alaris] (O.)
Levator labii superioris [m. quadratus labii superioris : caput infra-orbitale] (O.)
Levator anguli oris [caninus] (O.)
Zygomaticus minor [m. quadratus labii superioris : caput zygomaticum] (O.)
Zygomaticus major [zygomaticus] (O.)
Masseter (O. and I.)
Depressor alae nasi (O.)
Buccinator (O.)
Levator menti [mentalis] (O.)
Depressor labii inferioris [m. quadratus labii inferioris] (O.)
Depressor anguli oris [triangularis] (O.)
Platysma (O.)

Nasal bone
Orbital plate of ethmoid bone
Temporal line
Optic foramen
Parietal bone
Temporal surface of frontal bone
Zygomatic process of frontal
Superior orbital fissure
Greater wing of sphenoid bone
Temporal bone
Zygomatico-facial foramen
Zygomatic bone
Inferior orbital fissure
Maxilla
Mandibular notch
Mastoid process
Infra-orbital foramen (for infra-orbital vessels and nerve)
Middle concha of nose
Perpendicular plate of ethmoid
Inferior concha
Vomer
Mandible
Mental foramen for mental vessels and nerve
Symphysis menti

PLATE 23.—LATERAL ASPECT OF SKULL

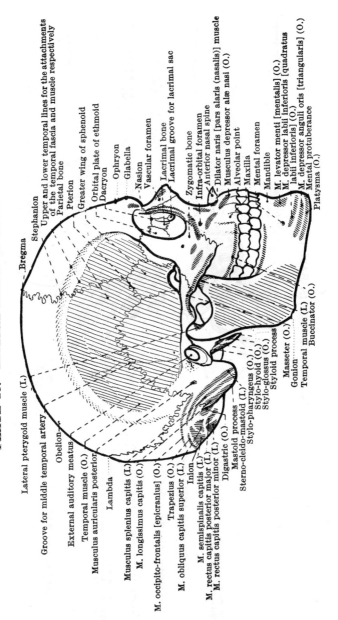

PLATE 24.—APERTURES IN BASE OF SKULL

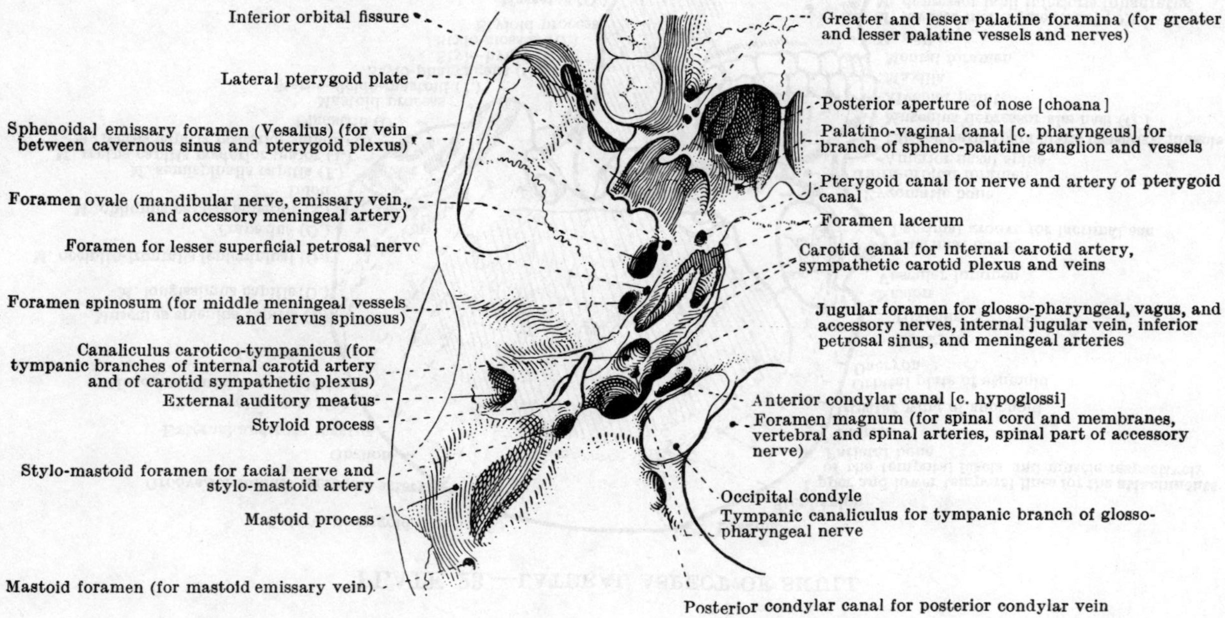

Labels (clockwise from top):

- Greater and lesser palatine foramina (for greater and lesser palatine vessels and nerves)
- Posterior aperture of nose [choana]
- Palatino-vaginal canal [c. pharyngeus] for branch of spheno-palatine ganglion and vessels
- Pterygoid canal for nerve and artery of pterygoid canal
- Foramen lacerum
- Carotid canal for internal carotid artery, sympathetic carotid plexus and veins
- Jugular foramen for glosso-pharyngeal, vagus, and accessory nerves, internal jugular vein, inferior petrosal sinus, and meningeal arteries
- Anterior condylar canal [c. hypoglossi]
- Foramen magnum (for spinal cord and membranes, vertebral and spinal arteries, spinal part of accessory nerve)
- Occipital condyle
- Tympanic canaliculus for tympanic branch of glosso-pharyngeal nerve
- Posterior condylar canal for posterior condylar vein

- Inferior orbital fissure
- Lateral pterygoid plate
- Sphenoidal emissary foramen (Vesalius) (for vein between cavernous sinus and pterygoid plexus)
- Foramen ovale (mandibular nerve, emissary vein, and accessory meningeal artery)
- Foramen for lesser superficial petrosal nerve
- Foramen spinosum (for middle meningeal vessels and nervus spinosus)
- Canaliculus carotico-tympanicus (for tympanic branches of internal carotid artery and of carotid sympathetic plexus)
- External auditory meatus
- Styloid process
- Stylo-mastoid foramen for facial nerve and stylo-mastoid artery
- Mastoid process
- Mastoid foramen (for mastoid emissary vein)

PLATE 25.—RIGHT ORBIT

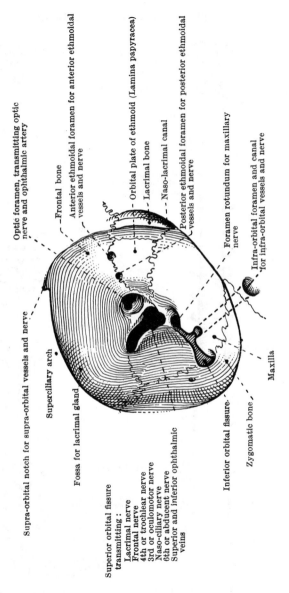

Optic foramen, transmitting optic nerve and ophthalmic artery

Frontal bone

Anterior ethmoidal foramen for anterior ethmoidal vessels and nerve

Orbital plate of ethmoid (Lamina papyracea)

Lacrimal bone

Naso-lacrimal canal

Posterior ethmoidal foramen for posterior ethmoidal vessels and nerve

Foramen rotundum for maxillary nerve

Infra-orbital foramen and canal for infra-orbital vessels and nerve

Supra-orbital notch for supra-orbital vessels and nerve

Superciliary arch

Fossa for lacrimal gland

Maxilla

Zygomatic bone

Inferior orbital fissure

Superior orbital fissure transmitting:
Lacrimal nerve
Frontal nerve
4th or trochlear nerve
3rd or oculomotor nerve
Naso-ciliary nerve
6th or abducent nerve
Superior and inferior ophthalmic veins

PLATE 26.—VERTEBRAL COLUMN

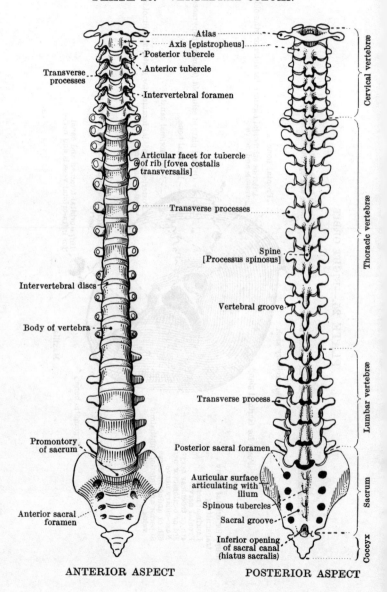

Atlas

Axis [epistropheus]

Posterior tubercle

Anterior tubercle

Intervertebral foramen

Transverse processes

Articular facet for tubercle of rib [fovea costalis transversalis]

Transverse processes

Spine [Processus spinosus]

Intervertebral discs

Vertebral groove

Body of vertebra

Transverse process

Promontory of sacrum

Posterior sacral foramen

Auricular surface articulating with ilium

Spinous tubercles

Sacral groove

Anterior sacral foramen

Inferior opening of sacral canal (hiatus sacralis)

Cervical vertebræ

Thoracic vertebræ

Lumbar vertebræ

Sacrum

Coccyx

ANTERIOR ASPECT

POSTERIOR ASPECT

PLATE 27.—VERTEBRAL COLUMN

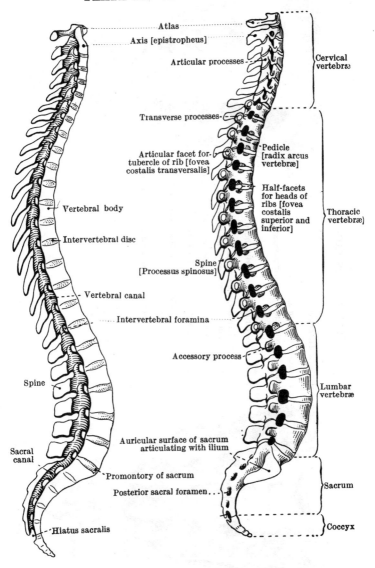

Atlas

Axis [epistropheus]

Articular processes

Cervical vertebræ

Transverse processes

Pedicle [radix arcus vertebræ]

Articular facet for tubercle of rib [fovea costalis transversalis]

Half-facets for heads of ribs [fovea costalis superior and inferior]

Vertebral body

Intervertebral disc

Spine [Processus spinosus]

Thoracic vertebræ

Vertebral canal

Intervertebral foramina

Accessory process

Spine

Lumbar vertebræ

Auricular surface of sacrum articulating with ilium

Sacral canal

Promontory of sacrum

Posterior sacral foramen

Sacrum

Hiatus sacralis

Coccyx

SECTION

LATERAL ASPECT

PLATE 28.—OS SACRUM

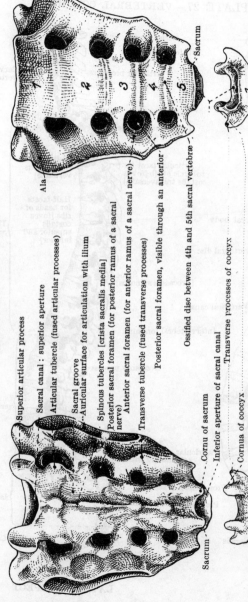

ANTERIOR ASPECT

POSTERIOR ASPECT

Superior articular process

Sacral canal : superior aperture

Articular tubercle (fused articular processes)

Sacral groove

Auricular surface for articulation with ilium

Spinous tubercles [crista sacralis media]

Posterior sacral foramen (for posterior ramus of a sacral nerve)

Anterior sacral foramen (for anterior ramus of a sacral nerve)

Transverse tubercle (fused transverse processes)

Posterior sacral foramen, visible through an anterior

Ossified disc between 4th and 5th sacral vertebræ

Transverse processes of coccyx

Cornu of sacrum

Inferior aperture of sacral canal

Cornua of coccyx

Ala.

Sacrum

Coccyx

Sacrum

Coccyx

PLATE 29.—OS SACRUM

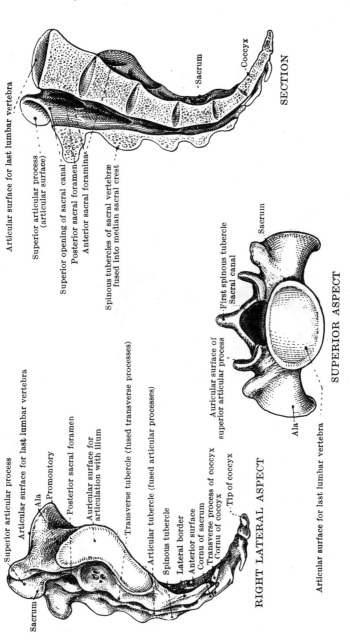

Articular surface for last lumbar vertebra

Superior articular process
(articular surface)

Superior opening of sacral canal
Posterior sacral foramen
Anterior sacral foramina

Spinous tubercles of sacral vertebrae
fused into median sacral crest

Sacrum

Coccyx

SECTION

Superior articular process

Ala
Promontory

Posterior sacral foramen

Auricular surface for
articulation with ilium

Transverse tubercle (fused transverse processes)

Articular tubercle (fused articular processes)

Spinous tubercle
Lateral border
Anterior surface
Cornu of sacrum
Transverse process of coccyx
Cornu of coccyx
Tip of coccyx

Auricular surface of
superior articular process

Sacrum

RIGHT LATERAL ASPECT

Articular surface for last lumbar vertebra

First spinous tubercle
Sacral canal

Sacrum

Ala

Articular surface for last lumbar vertebra

SUPERIOR ASPECT

PLATE 30.—ATLAS (1st CERVICAL) VERTEBRA

SUPERIOR ASPECT

Vertebral foramen
1st cervical spinal nerve
Vertebral artery
Transverse process
Posterior tubercle
Posterior arch
Foramen for vertebral artery (foramen transversarium)
Superior articular surface for condyle of occipital bone
Facet for odontoid process [fovea dentis]
Tubercle for attachment of transverse ligament
Anterior arch
Anterior tubercle
Vertebral foramen
Posterior arch,
Anterior arch
Inferior articular surface, for superior articular surface of axis [epistropheus]

INFERIOR ASPECT

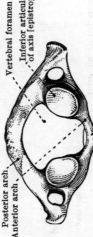

Course of the vertebral artery
Anterior arch
Transverse process

RIGHT LATERAL ASPECT

Posterior arch,
Anterior arch,
Transverse process
Lateral masses

ANTERIOR ASPECT

Anterior arch Posterior arch
Superior articular surface,
Foramen for vertebral artery (foramen transversarium)
Transverse process

PLATE 31.—AXIS (2ND CERVICAL) VERTEBRA [EPISTROPHEUS]

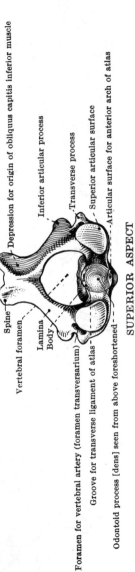

Spine — Depression for origin of obliquus capitis inferior muscle

Inferior articular process

Transverse process

Superior articular surface

Articular surface for anterior arch of atlas

Foramen for vertebral artery (foramen transversarium)

Groove for transverse ligament of atlas

Lamina

Body

Vertebral foramen

Odontoid process [dens] seen from above foreshortened

SUPERIOR ASPECT

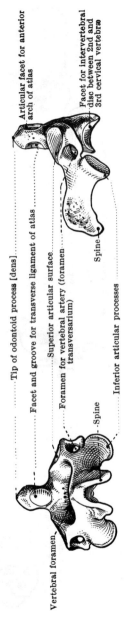

Articular facet for anterior arch of atlas

Facet for intervertebral disc between 2nd and 3rd cervical vertebræ

Spine

RIGHT LATERAL ASPECT

Tip of odontoid process [dens]

Facet and groove for transverse ligament of atlas

Superior articular surface

Foramen for vertebral artery (foramen transversarium)

Inferior articular processes

Spine

Vertebral foramen

POSTERIOR ASPECT

PLATE 32.—CERVICAL, THORACIC, AND LUMBAR VERTEBRÆ

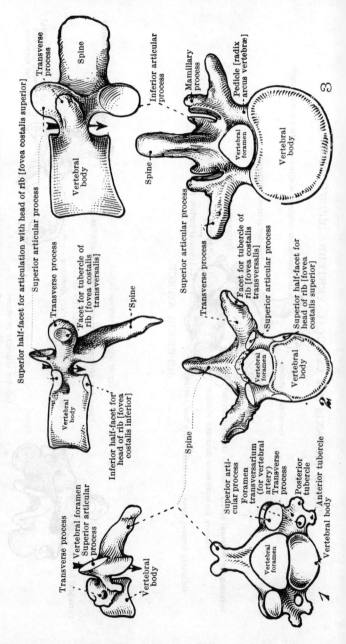

Superior half-facet for articulation with head of rib [fovea costalis superior]

Transverse process

Spine

Inferior articular process

Mamillary process

Pedicle [radix arcus vertebræ]

Vertebral foramen

Vertebral body

Spine

Superior articular process

Transverse process

Facet for tubercle of rib [fovea costalis transversalis]

Inferior half-facet for head of rib [fovea costalis inferior]

Spine

Superior articular process

Transverse process

Facet for tubercle of rib [fovea costalis transversalis]

Superior articular process

Superior half-facet for head of rib [fovea costalis superior]

Vertebral foramen

Vertebral body

Spine

Vertebral foramen

Superior articular process

Vertebral body

Transverse process

Vertebral foramen

Superior articular process

Vertebral body

Superior articular process

Foramen transversarium (for vertebral artery)

Transverse process

Posterior tubercle

Anterior tubercle

Vertebral foramen

Vertebral body

3

PLATE 33

ORIGIN AND EMERGENCE OF ROOTS OF SPINAL NERVES

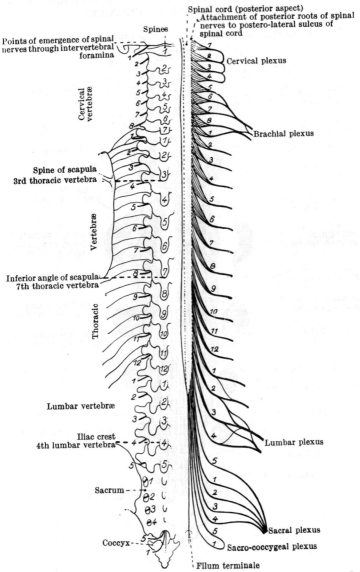

Spinal cord (posterior aspect)

Attachment of posterior roots of spinal nerves to postero-lateral sulcus of spinal cord

Spines

Points of emergence of spinal nerves through intervertebral foramina

Cervical vertebræ

Cervical plexus

Brachial plexus

Spine of scapula
3rd thoracic vertebra

Vertebræ

Inferior angle of scapula
7th thoracic vertebra

Thoracic

Lumbar vertebræ

Iliac crest
4th lumbar vertebra

Lumbar plexus

Sacrum

Sacral plexus

Coccyx

Sacro-coccygeal plexus

Filum terminale

3

PLATE 34.—SPINAL NERVE ROOTS IN THE SACRAL CANAL
(PARTLY AFTER HOVELACQUE)

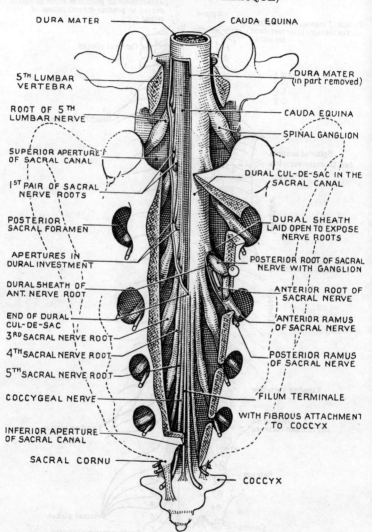

DURA MATER

CAUDA EQUINA

5TH LUMBAR VERTEBRA

DURA MATER (in part removed)

ROOT OF 5TH LUMBAR NERVE

CAUDA EQUINA

SPINAL GANGLION

SUPERIOR APERTURE OF SACRAL CANAL

1ST PAIR OF SACRAL NERVE ROOTS

DURAL CUL-DE-SAC IN THE SACRAL CANAL

POSTERIOR SACRAL FORAMEN

DURAL SHEATH LAID OPEN TO EXPOSE NERVE ROOTS

APERTURES IN DURAL INVESTMENT

POSTERIOR ROOT OF SACRAL NERVE WITH GANGLION

DURAL SHEATH OF ANT. NERVE ROOT

ANTERIOR ROOT OF SACRAL NERVE

END OF DURAL CUL-DE-SAC

ANTERIOR RAMUS OF SACRAL NERVE

3RD SACRAL NERVE ROOT

4TH SACRAL NERVE ROOT

POSTERIOR RAMUS OF SACRAL NERVE

5TH SACRAL NERVE ROOT

COCCYGEAL NERVE

FILUM TERMINALE

WITH FIBROUS ATTACHMENT TO COCCYX

INFERIOR APERTURE OF SACRAL CANAL

SACRAL CORNU

COCCYX

PLATE 35.—SPINAL CORD [MEDULLA] AND MENINGES

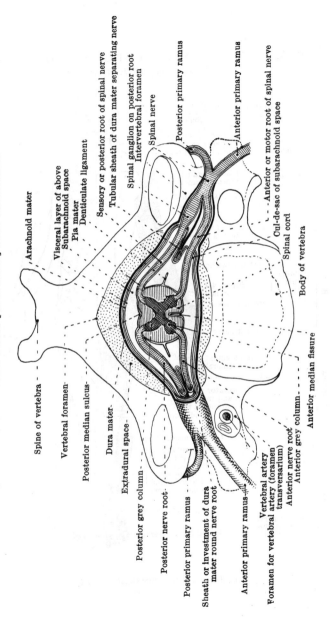

Spine of vertebra

Vertebral foramen

Posterior median sulcus

Dura mater

Extradural space

Posterior grey column

Posterior nerve root

Sheath or investment of dura
mater round nerve root

Anterior primary ramus

Vertebral artery
Foramen for vertebral artery (foramen
transversarium)
Anterior nerve root
Anterior grey column

Anterior median fissure

Arachnoid mater

Visceral layer of above
Subarachnoid space
Pia mater
Denticulate ligament

Sensory or posterior root of spinal nerve
Tubular sheath of dura mater separating nerve

Spinal ganglion on posterior root
Intervertebral foramen

Spinal nerve

Posterior primary ramus

Anterior primary ramus

Anterior or motor root of spinal nerve

Cul-de-sac of subarachnoid space

Spinal cord

Body of vertebra

PLATE 36.—PERIPHERAL DISTRIBUTION OF SENSORY NERVES—ANTERIOR ASPECT

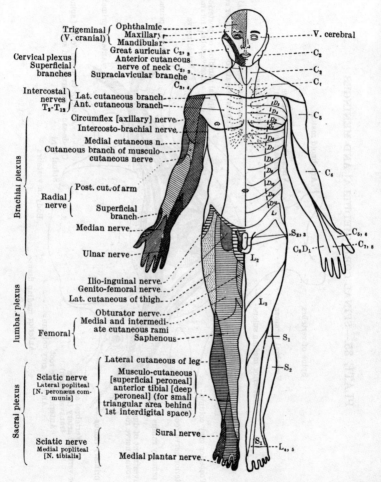

Trigeminal (V. cranial) { Ophthalmic
Maxillary
Mandibular

V. cerebral

Cervical plexus Superficial branches { Great auricular C$_{2, 3}$
Anterior cutaneous nerve of neck C$_{2, 3}$
Supraclavicular branche C$_{3, 4}$

C$_2$

C$_3$

C$_4$

Intercostal nerves T$_2$-T$_{12}$ { Lat. cutaneous branch
Ant. cutaneous branch

C$_5$

Circumflex [axillary] nerve
Intercosto-brachial nerve
Medial cutaneous n.
Cutaneous branch of musculo-cutaneous nerve

D$_2$
D$_3$
D$_4$
D$_5$
D$_6$
D$_7$
D$_8$
D$_9$

C$_6$

Radial nerve { Post. cut. of arm
Superficial branch

D$_{10}$
D$_{11}$
D$_{12}$
L$_1$

Median nerve

S$_{2, 3}$

C$_{5, 6}$

Ulnar nerve

L$_2$

C$_8$D$_1$

C$_{7, 8}$

Ilio-inguinal nerve
Genito-femoral nerve
Lat. cutaneous of thigh

L$_3$

Femoral { Obturator nerve
Medial and intermediate cutaneous rami
Saphenous

S$_1$

Sciatic nerve Lateral popliteal [N. peronæus communis] { Lateral cutaneous of leg
Musculo-cutaneous [superficial peroneal] anterior tibial [deep peroneal] (for small triangular area behind 1st interdigital space)

S$_2$

Sciatic nerve Medial popliteal [N. tibialis] { Sural nerve
Medial plantar nerve

S$_1$

L$_{4, 5}$

Brachial plexus

lumbar plexus

Sacral plexus

D$_2$, D$_3$, etc., in the figure signify *Thoracic*$_2$, etc.

PLATE 37.—PERIPHERAL DISTRIBUTION OF SENSORY NERVES—POSTERIOR ASPECT

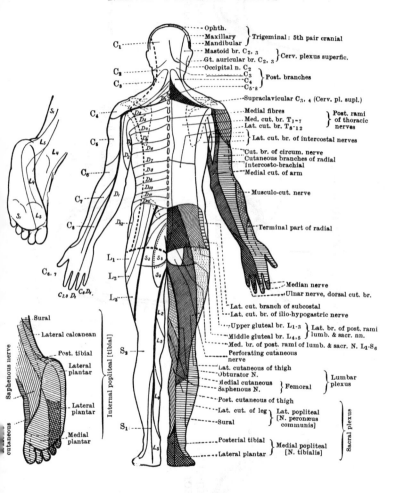

D$_2$, D$_3$. etc., in the figure signify *Thoracic*$_2$, etc.

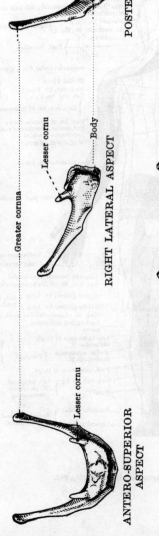
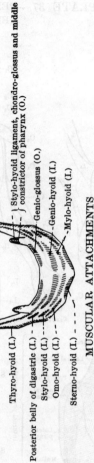

PLATE 38.—HYOID BONE

ANTERO-SUPERIOR ASPECT

Lesser cornu

Greater cornu

Lesser cornu

Body

RIGHT LATERAL ASPECT

POSTERO-INFERIOR ASPECT

MUSCULAR ATTACHMENTS

Middle constrictor of pharynx (O.)

Stylo-hyoid ligament, chondro-glossus and middle constrictor of pharynx (O.)

Genio-glossus (O.)

Genio-hyoid (I.)

Mylo-hyoid (I.)

Hyo-glossus

Thyro-hyoid (I.)

Posterior belly of digastric (I.)

Stylo-hyoid (I.)

Omo-hyoid (I.)

Sterno-hyoid (I.)

PLATE 39.—CLAVICLE—COLLAR BONE

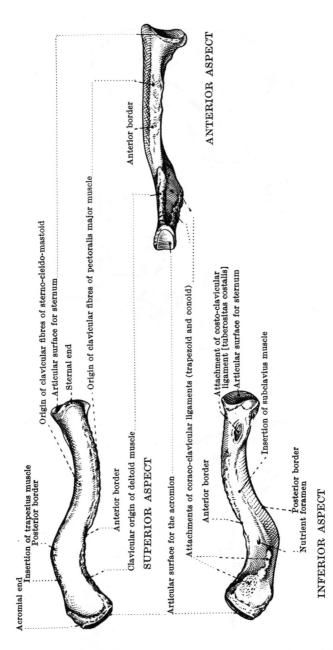

ANTERIOR ASPECT

Anterior border

Origin of clavicular fibres of pectoralis major muscle

Sternal end

Articular surface for sternum

Origin of clavicular fibres of sterno-cleido-mastoid

Insertion of trapezius muscle

Posterior border

Acromial end

Anterior border

Clavicular origin of deltoid muscle

SUPERIOR ASPECT

Articular surface for the acromion

Attachments of coraco-clavicular ligaments (trapezoid and conoid)

Anterior border

Attachment of costo-clavicular ligament [tuberositas costalis]

Articular surface for sternum

Insertion of subclavius muscle

Posterior border

Nutrient foramen

INFERIOR ASPECT

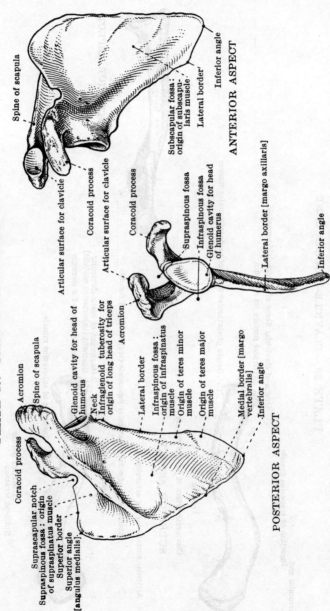

PLATE 40.—SCAPULA—SHOULDER BLADE

Spine of scapula

Articular surface for clavicle

Coracoid process

Subscapular fossa:
origin of subscapu-
laris muscle

Lateral border

Inferior angle

ANTERIOR ASPECT

Coracoid process

Articular surface for clavicle

Coracoid process

Supraspinous fossa

Infraspinous fossa

Glenoid cavity for head
of humerus

Lateral border [margo axillaris]

Inferior angle

LATERAL ASPECT

Coracoid process

Acromion

Spine of scapula

Glenoid cavity for head of
humerus

Neck

Infraglenoid tuberosity for
origin of long head of triceps

Acromion

Lateral border

Infraspinous fossa:
origin of infraspinatus
muscle

Origin of teres minor
muscle

Origin of teres major
muscle

Medial border [margo
vertebralis]

Inferior angle

Suprascapular notch
Supraspinous fossa : origin
of supraspinatus muscle
Superior border
Superior angle
[angulus medialis]

Coracoid process

POSTERIOR ASPECT

PLATE 41.—STERNUM—BREAST BONE

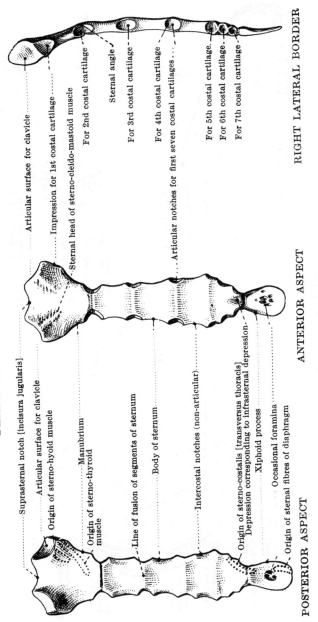

RIGHT LATERAL BORDER

Articular surface for clavicle
Impression for 1st costal cartilage
Sternal head of sterno-cleido-mastoid muscle
For 2nd costal cartilage
Sternal angle
For 3rd costal cartilage
For 4th costal cartilage
Articular notches for first seven costal cartilages
For 5th costal cartilage.
For 6th costal cartilage.
For 7th costal cartilage

ANTERIOR ASPECT

Suprasternal notch [incisura jugularis]
Articular surface for clavicle
Origin of sterno-hyoid muscle
Manubrium
Origin of sterno-thyroid muscle
Line of fusion of segments of sternum
Body of sternum
Intercostal notches (non-articular)
Origin of sterno-costalis [transversus thoracis]
Depression corresponding to infrasternal depression
Xiphoid process
Occasional foramina
Origin of sternal fibres of diaphragm

POSTERIOR ASPECT

PLATE 42.—COSTÆ—THE RIBS

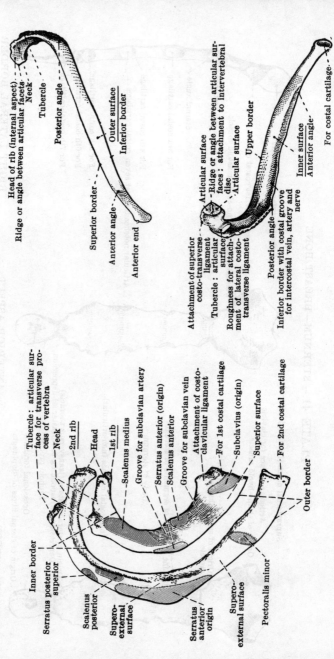

PLATE 43.—THE THORACIC CAGE

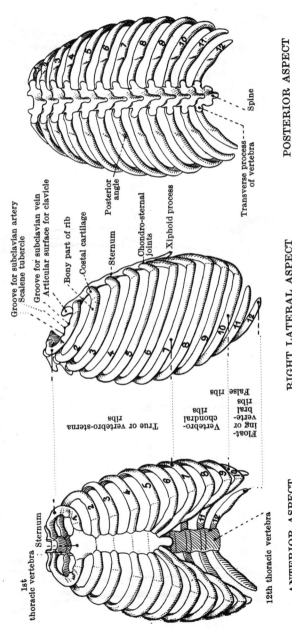

ANTERIOR ASPECT

RIGHT LATERAL ASPECT

POSTERIOR ASPECT

1st thoracic vertebra

Sternum

12th thoracic vertebra

Groove for subclavian artery
Scalene tubercle
Groove for subclavian vein
Articular surface for clavicle
Bony part of rib
Costal cartilage
Sternum
Posterior angle
Chondro-sternal joints
Xiphoid process

Spine
Transverse process of vertebra

True or vertebro-sterna ribs

Vertebro-chondral ribs
Float-ing or vertebral ribs
False ribs

PLATE 44.—HUMERUS

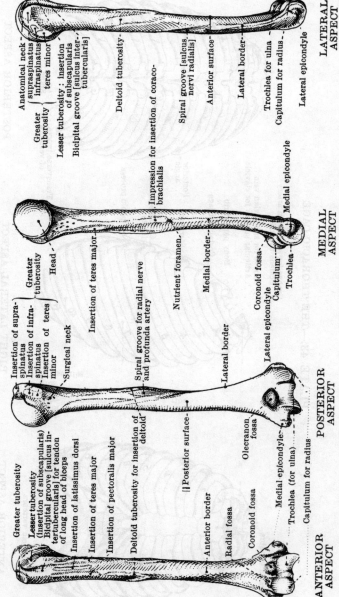

LATERAL ASPECT

Anatomical neck
Greater tuberosity { supraspinatus · infraspinatus · teres minor
Lesser tuberosity : Insertion of subscapularis
Bicipital groove [sulcus intertubercularis]
Deltoid tuberosity
Spiral groove [sulcus nervi radialis]
Anterior surface
Lateral border
Trochlea for ulna
Capitulum for radius
Lateral epicondyle

MEDIAL ASPECT

Head
Greater tuberosity
Insertion of teres major
Impression for insertion of coracobrachialis
Nutrient foramen
Medial border
Coronoid fossa
Lateral epicondyle
Capitulum
Trochlea
Medial epicondyle

POSTERIOR ASPECT

Insertion of supraspinatus
Insertion of infraspinatus
Insertion of teres minor
Surgical neck
Spiral groove for radial nerve and profunda artery
Lateral border
Medial epicondyle
Olecranon fossa
|| Posterior surface

ANTERIOR ASPECT

Greater tuberosity
Lesser tuberosity (Insertion of subscapularis)
Bicipital groove [sulcus intertubercularis] for tendon of long head of biceps
Insertion of latissimus dorsi
Insertion of teres major
Insertion of pectoralis major
Deltoid tuberosity for insertion of deltoid
Anterior border
Radial fossa
Coronoid fossa
Medial epicondyle
Trochlea (for ulna)
Capitulum for radius

PLATE 45.—ULNA AND RADIUS

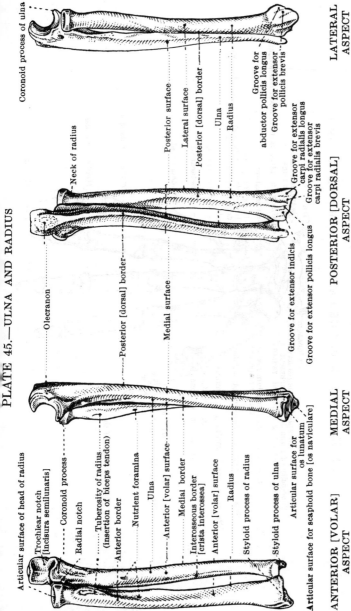

Coronoid process of ulna

Neck of radius

Posterior surface

Lateral surface

Posterior [dorsal] border

Ulna

Radius

Groove for abductor pollicis longus

Groove for extensor pollicis brevis

Groove for extensor carpi radialis longus

Groove for extensor carpi radialis brevis

Groove for extensor indicis

Groove for extensor pollicis longus

Articular surface of head of radius

Trochlear notch [incisura semilunaris]

Coronoid process

Radial notch

Tuberosity of radius (insertion of biceps tendon)

Anterior border

Nutrient foramina

Ulna

Anterior [volar] surface

Medial border

Interosseous border [crista interossea]

Anterior [volar] surface

Radius

Styloid process of radius

Styloid process of ulna

Articular surface for os lunatum [os naviculare]

Articular surface for scaphoid bone [os naviculare]

Olecranon

Posterior [dorsal] border

Medial surface

LATERAL ASPECT

POSTERIOR [DORSAL] ASPECT

MEDIAL ASPECT

ANTERIOR [VOLAR] ASPECT

PLATE 46.—BONES OF THE HAND—PALMAR [VOLAR] ASPECT

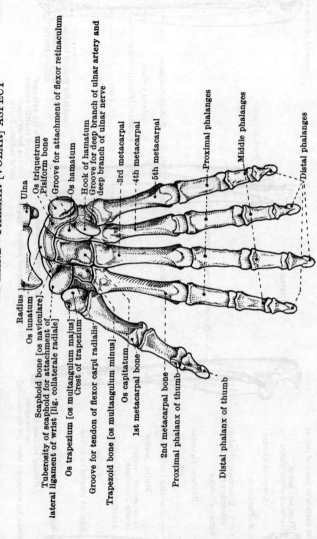

Radius
Ulna
Os lunatum
Os triquetrum
Pisiform bone
Scaphoid bone [os naviculare]
Groove for attachment of flexor retinaculum
Tuberosity of scaphoid for attachment of
lateral ligament of wrist [lig. collaterale radiale]
Os hamatum
Os trapezium [os multangulum majus]
Crest of trapezium
Hook of hamatum
Groove for deep branch of ulnar artery and
deep branch of ulnar nerve
Groove for tendon of flexor carpi radialis
3rd metacarpal
Trapezoid bone [os multangulum minus]
4th metacarpal
Os capitatum
5th metacarpal
1st metacarpal bone
Proximal phalanges
2nd metacarpal bone
Proximal phalanx of thumb
Middle phalanges
Distal phalanges
Distal phalanx of thumb

PLATE 47.—BONES OF THE HAND—DORSAL ASPECT

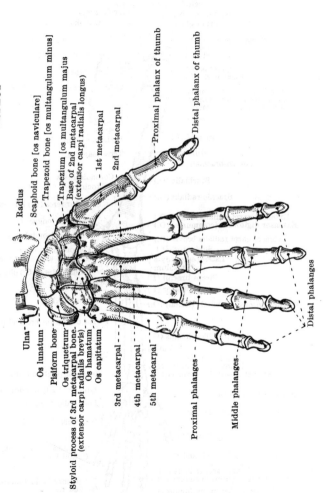

Ulna
Radius
Os lunatum
Scaphoid bone [os naviculare]
Pisiform bone
Trapezoid bone [os multangulum minus]
Os triquetrum
Trapezium [os multangulum majus]
Styloid process of 3rd metacarpal bone
(extensor carpi radialis brevis)
Base of 2nd metacarpal
(extensor carpi radialis longus)
Os hamatum
1st metacarpal
Os capitatum
2nd metacarpal

3rd metacarpal
4th metacarpal
5th metacarpal

Proximal phalanx of thumb
Distal phalanx of thumb

Proximal phalanges
Middle phalanges
Distal phalanges

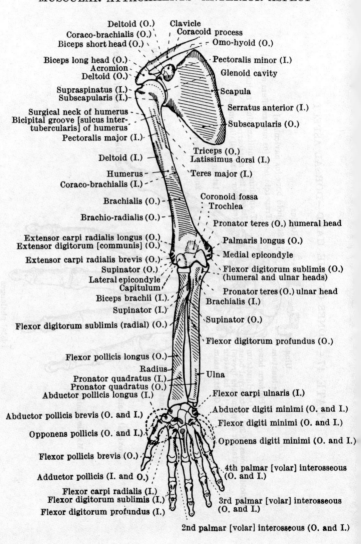

Deltoid (O.)
Coraco-brachialis (O.)
Biceps short head (O.)
Clavicle
Coracoid process
Omo-hyoid (O.)
Biceps long head (O.)
Acromion
Deltoid (O.)
Pectoralis minor (I.)
Glenoid cavity
Supraspinatus (I.)
Subscapularis (I.)
Scapula
Serratus anterior (I.)
Surgical neck of humerus
Bicipital groove [sulcus inter-tubercularis] of humerus
Subscapularis (O.)
Pectoralis major (I.)
Deltoid (I.)
Triceps (O.)
Latissimus dorsi (I.)
Humerus
Coraco-brachialis (I.)
Teres major (I.)
Brachialis (O.)
Coronoid fossa
Trochlea
Brachio-radialis (O.)
Pronator teres (O.) humeral head
Extensor carpi radialis longus (O.)
Extensor digitorum [communis] (O.)
Palmaris longus (O.)
Medial epicondyle
Extensor carpi radialis brevis (O.)
Supinator (I.)
Lateral epicondyle
Capitulum
Flexor digitorum sublimis (O.) (humeral and ulnar heads)
Biceps brachii (I.)
Supinator (I.)
Pronator teres (O.) ulnar head
Brachialis (I.)
Flexor digitorum sublimis (radial) (O.)
Supinator (O.)
Flexor digitorum profundus (O.)
Flexor pollicis longus (O.)
Radius
Pronator quadratus (I.)
Pronator quadratus (O.)
Abductor pollicis longus (I.)
Ulna
Flexor carpi ulnaris (I.)
Abductor pollicis brevis (O. and I.)
Abductor digiti minimi (O. and I.)
Flexor digiti minimi (O. and I.)
Opponens pollicis (O. and I.)
Opponens digiti minimi (O. and I.)
Flexor pollicis brevis (O.)
4th palmar [volar] interosseous (O. and I.)
Adductor pollicis (I. and O.)
Flexor carpi radialis (I.)
Flexor digitorum sublimis (I.)
Flexor digitorum profundus (I.)
3rd palmar [volar] interosseous (O. and I.)
2nd palmar [volar] interosseous (O. and I.)

PLATE 49.—BONES OF THE UPPER LIMB, SHOWING
MUSCULAR ATTACHMENTS—POSTERIOR ASPECT

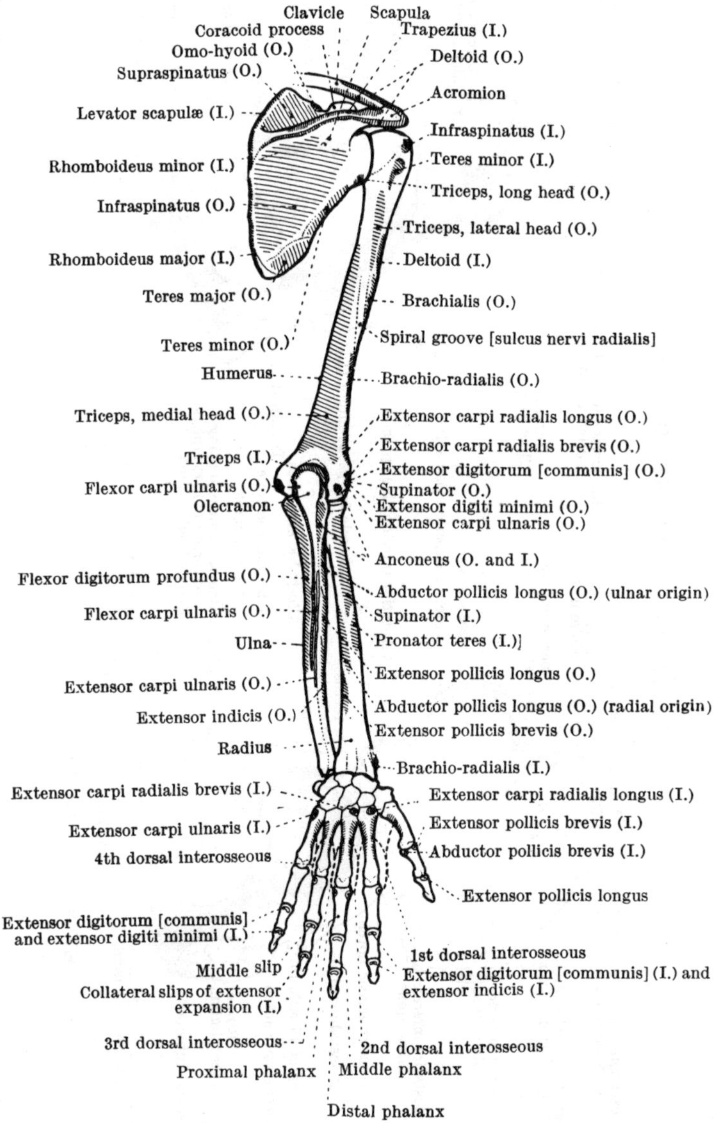

Clavicle
Coracoid process
Omo-hyoid (O.)
Supraspinatus (O.)
Levator scapulæ (I.)
Rhomboideus minor (I.)
Infraspinatus (O.)
Rhomboideus major (I.)
Teres major (O.)
Teres minor (O.)
Humerus
Triceps, medial head (O.)
Triceps (I.)
Flexor carpi ulnaris (O.)
Olecranon
Flexor digitorum profundus (O.)
Flexor carpi ulnaris (O.)
Ulna
Extensor carpi ulnaris (O.)
Extensor indicis (O.)
Radius
Extensor carpi radialis brevis (I.)
Extensor carpi ulnaris (I.)
4th dorsal interosseous
Extensor digitorum [communis]
and extensor digiti minimi (I.)
Middle slip
Collateral slips of extensor
expansion (I.)
3rd dorsal interosseous
Proximal phalanx

Scapula
Trapezius (I.)
Deltoid (O.)
Acromion
Infraspinatus (I.)
Teres minor (I.)
Triceps, long head (O.)
Triceps, lateral head (O.)
Deltoid (I.)
Brachialis (O.)
Spiral groove [sulcus nervi radialis]
Brachio-radialis (O.)
Extensor carpi radialis longus (O.)
Extensor carpi radialis brevis (O.)
Extensor digitorum [communis] (O.)
Supinator (O.)
Extensor digiti minimi (O.)
Extensor carpi ulnaris (O.)
Anconeus (O. and I.)
Abductor pollicis longus (O.) (ulnar origin)
Supinator (I.)
Pronator teres (I.)]
Extensor pollicis longus (O.)
Abductor pollicis longus (O.) (radial origin)
Extensor pollicis brevis (O.)
Brachio-radialis (I.)
Extensor carpi radialis longus (I.)
Extensor pollicis brevis (I.)
Abductor pollicis brevis (I.)
Extensor pollicis longus
1st dorsal interosseous
Extensor digitorum [communis] (I.) and
extensor indicis (I.)
2nd dorsal interosseous
Middle phalanx

Distal phalanx

4

PLATE 50.—HIP BONE—OS COXÆ

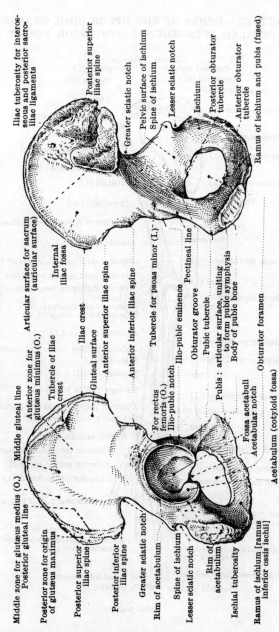

Internal aspect (labels, top):
Iliac tuberosity for interosseous and posterior sacroiliac ligaments
Posterior superior iliac spine
Greater sciatic notch
Pelvic surface of ischium
Spine of ischium
Lesser sciatic notch
Ischium
Posterior obturator tubercle
Anterior obturator tubercle
Ramus of ischium and pubis (fused)
Articular surface for sacrum (auricular surface)
Internal iliac fossa
Tuber for psoas minor (L.)
Pectineal line
Pubis: articular surface, uniting to form pubic symphysis
Body of pubic bone
Obturator groove
Pubic tubercle
Ilio-pubic eminence
Anterior inferior iliac spine
Anterior superior iliac spine
Iliac crest
Tubercle of iliac crest
Anterior zone for gluteus minimus (O.)
Middle gluteal line

INTERNAL ASPECT

External aspect (labels, bottom):
Middle zone for gluteus medius (O.)
Posterior gluteal line
Posterior zone for origin of gluteus maximus
Posterior superior iliac spine
Posterior inferior iliac spine
Greater sciatic notch
Spine of ischium
Lesser sciatic notch
Ischial tuberosity
Ramus of ischium [ramus inferior ossis ischii]
Acetabulum (cotyloid fossa)
Fossa acetabuli
Acetabular notch
Rim of acetabulum
Ilio-pubic notch
For rectus femoris (O.)
Anterior inferior iliac spine
Anterior superior iliac spine
Gluteal surface
Tubercle of iliac crest
Iliac crest
Obturator foramen
Obturator groove
Ilio-pubic eminence
Pectineal line

EXTERNAL ASPECT

PLATE 51.—FEMUR—THIGH BONE

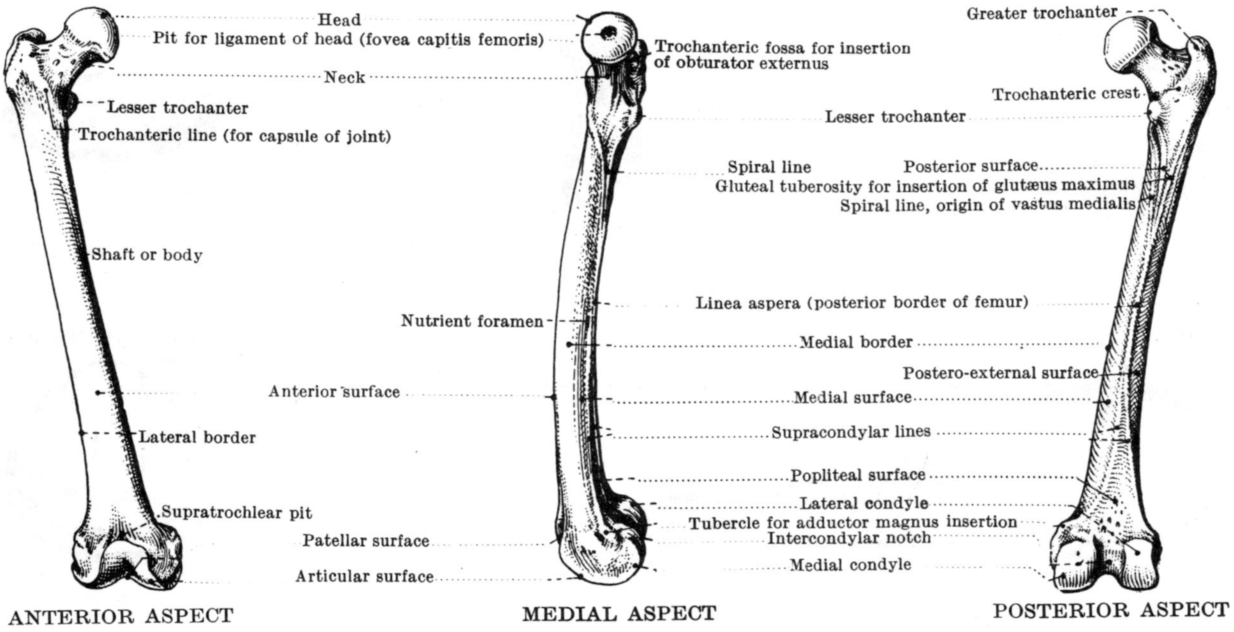

Greater trochanter

Trochanteric crest

Trochanteric fossa for insertion of obturator externus

Lesser trochanter

Posterior surface

Gluteal tuberosity for insertion of gluteus maximus

Spiral line, origin of vastus medialis

Spiral line

Linea aspera (posterior border of femur)

Medial border

Postero-external surface

Medial surface

Supracondylar lines

Popliteal surface

Lateral condyle

Tubercle for adductor magnus insertion

Intercondylar notch

Medial condyle

POSTERIOR ASPECT

Head

Pit for ligament of head (fovea capitis femoris)

Neck

Trochanteric line (for capsule of joint)

Nutrient foramen

Anterior surface

Supratrochlear pit

Patellar surface

Articular surface

MEDIAL ASPECT

Lesser trochanter

Shaft or body

Lateral border

ANTERIOR ASPECT

PLATE 52.—PATELLA—KNEE CAP

Facet for lateral condyle of femur

Posterior or articular surface

Facet corresponding with (in flexion) the lateral border of medial condyle

Articular facet for medial condyle

Non-articular portion in relation with infrapatellar pad of fat.

POSTERIOR ASPECT

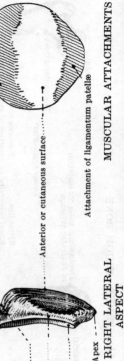

Insertion of quadriceps femoris

Anterior or cutaneous surface

Attachment of ligamentum patellæ

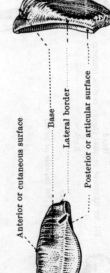

MUSCULAR ATTACHMENTS

Lateral border

Base or superior border

Medial border

Anterior or cutaneous surface

Apex

ANTERIOR ASPECT

Anterior or cutaneous surface

Base

Lateral border

Posterior or articular surface

Apex

RIGHT LATERAL ASPECT

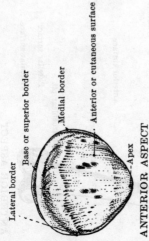

SUPERIOR ASPECT

PLATE 53.—TIBIA AND FIBULA

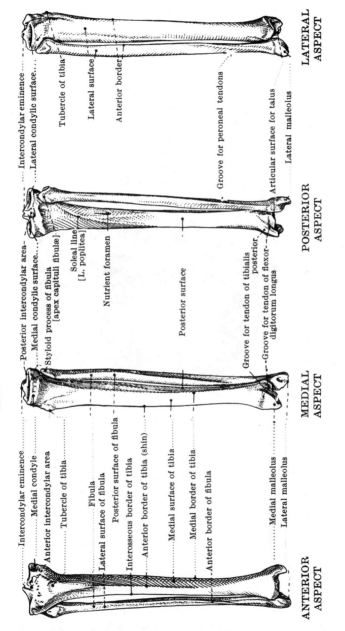

Intercondylar eminence

Lateral condylic surface

Tubercle of tibia

Lateral surface

Anterior border

Groove for peroneal tendons

Articular surface for talus

Lateral malleolus

LATERAL ASPECT

Intercondylar eminence

Posterior intercondylar area

Medial condylic surface

Styloid process of fibula [apex capituli fibulæ]

Soleal line [L. popliteal]

Nutrient foramen

Posterior surface

Groove for tendon of tibialis posterior

Groove for tendon of flexor digitorum longus

POSTERIOR ASPECT

Groove for tendon of tibialis posterior

Groove for tendon of flexor digitorum longus

MEDIAL ASPECT

Intercondylar eminence

Medial condyle

Anterior intercondylar area

Tubercle of tibia

Fibula

Lateral surface of fibula

Posterior surface of fibula

Interosseous border of tibia

Anterior border of tibia (shin)

Medial surface of tibia

Medial border of tibia

Anterior border of fibula

Medial malleolus

Lateral malleolus

ANTERIOR ASPECT

PLATE 54.—TRANSVERSE SECTION OF LEG AT LEVEL OF MALLEOLI

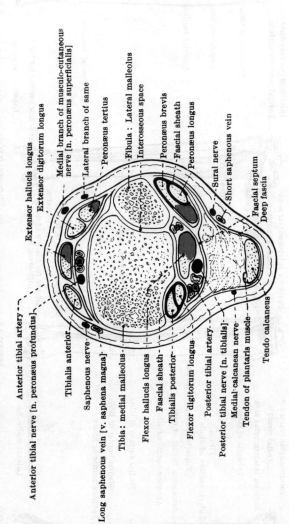

Anterior tibial artery
Anterior tibial nerve [n. peronæus profundus]
Extensor hallucis longus
Extensor digitorum longus
Medial branch of musculo-cutaneous nerve [n. peronæus superficialis]
Lateral branch of same
Peronæus tertius
Fibula : Lateral malleolus
Interosseous space
Peronæus brevis
Fascial sheath
Peronæus longus
Sural nerve
Short saphenous vein
Fascial septum
Deep fascia

Tibialis anterior
Saphenous nerve
Long saphenous vein [v. saphena magna]
Tibia : medial malleolus
Flexor hallucis longus
Fascial sheath
Tibialis posterior
Flexor digitorum longus
Posterior tibial artery
Posterior tibial nerve [n. tibialis]
Medial calcanean nerve
Tendon of plantaris muscle
Tendo calcaneus

PLATE 55.—BONES OF THE FOOT

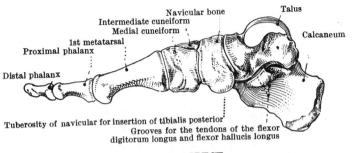

Navicular bone

Intermediate cuneiform
Medial cuneiform

1st metatarsal

Proximal phalanx

Distal phalanx

Talus

Calcaneum

Tuberosity of navicular for insertion of tibialis posterior

Grooves for the tendons of the flexor
digitorum longus and flexor hallucis longus

MEDIAL ASPECT

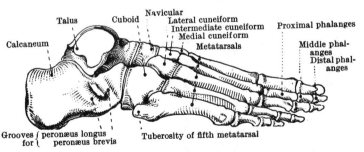

Talus   Cuboid   Navicular
                         Lateral cuneiform
                         Intermediate cuneiform
                         Medial cuneiform

Calcaneum   Metatarsals

Proximal phalanges

Middle phal-
anges
Distal phal-
anges

Grooves ⎰ peronæus longus
for   ⎱ peronæus brevis   Tuberosity of fifth metatarsal

LATERAL ASPECT

PLATE 56.—BONES OF THE FOOT—DORSAL ASPECT

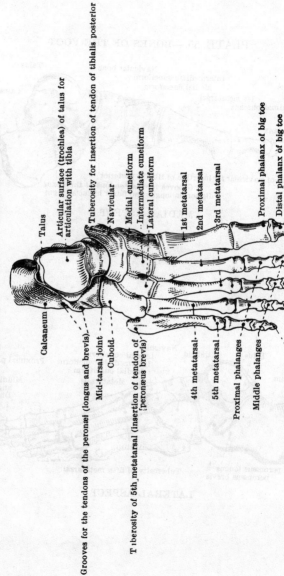

- Talus
- Articular surface (trochlea) of talus for articulation with tibia
- Tuberosity for insertion of tendon of tibialis posterior
- Navicular
- Medial cuneiform
- Intermediate cuneiform
- Lateral cuneiform
- 1st metatarsal
- 2nd metatarsal
- 3rd metatarsal
- Proximal phalanx of big toe
- Distal phalanx of big toe

- Calcaneum
- Grooves for the tendons of the peronæi (longus and brevis)
- Mid-tarsal joint
- Cuboid
- Tuberosity of 5th metatarsal (insertion of tendon of peronæus brevis)
- 4th metatarsal
- 5th metatarsal
- Proximal phalanges
- Middle phalanges
- Distal phalanges

PLATE 57.—BONES OF THE FOOT—PLANTAR ASPECT

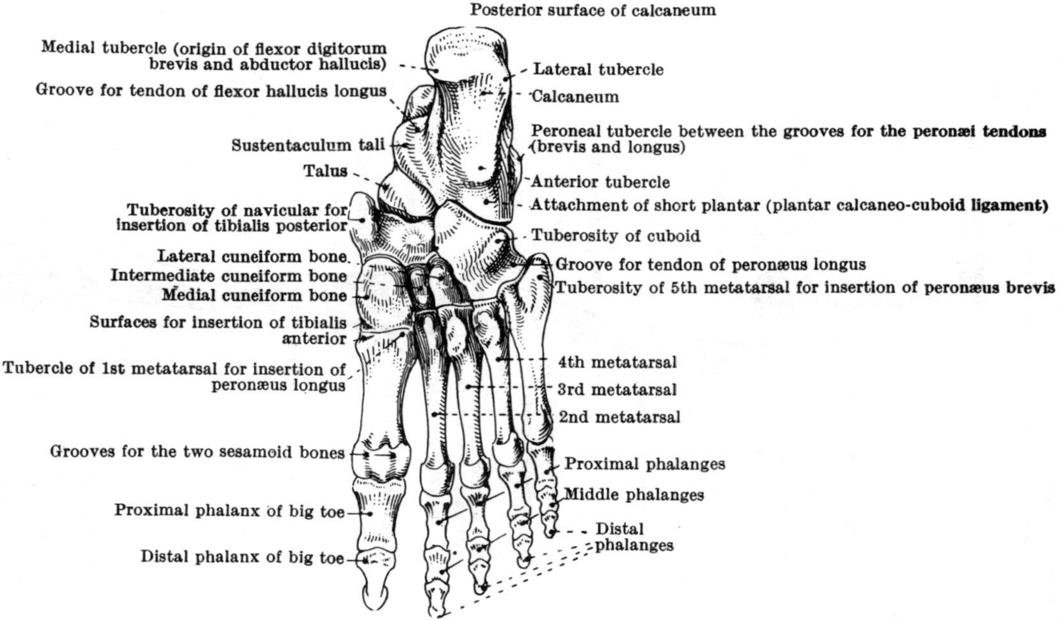

Posterior surface of calcaneum

Lateral tubercle

Calcaneum

Peroneal tubercle between the grooves for the peronaei tendons (brevis and longus)

Anterior tubercle

Attachment of short plantar (plantar calcaneo-cuboid ligament)

Tuberosity of cuboid

Groove for tendon of peroneus longus

Tuberosity of 5th metatarsal for insertion of peroneus brevis

4th metatarsal

3rd metatarsal

2nd metatarsal

Proximal phalanges

Middle phalanges

Distal phalanges

Medial tubercle (origin of flexor digitorum brevis and abductor hallucis)

Groove for tendon of flexor hallucis longus

Sustentaculum tali

Talus

Tuberosity of navicular for insertion of tibialis posterior

Lateral cuneiform bone

Intermediate cuneiform bone

Medial cuneiform bone

Surfaces for insertion of tibialis anterior

Tubercle of 1st metatarsal for insertion of peroneus longus

Grooves for the two sesamoid bones

Proximal phalanx of big toe

Distal phalanx of big toe

PLATE 58.—BONES OF THE LOWER LIMB, SHOWING MUSCULAR ATTACHMENTS—ANTERIOR ASPECT

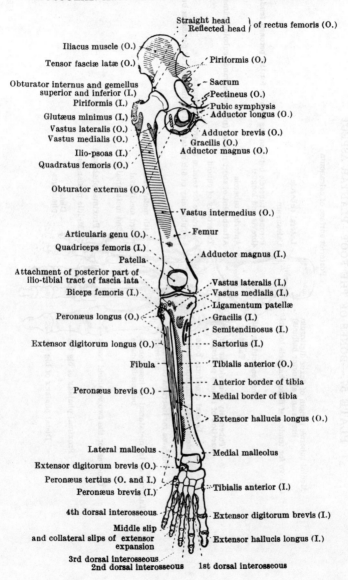

Straight head
Reflected head } of rectus femoris (O.)

Iliacus muscle (O.)

Tensor fasciæ latæ (O.)

Piriformis (O.)

Obturator internus and gemellus
superior and inferior (I.)

Sacrum

Pectineus (O.)

Piriformis (I.)

Pubic symphysis

Glutæus minimus (I.)

Adductor longus (O.)

Vastus lateralis (O.)

Vastus medialis (O.)

Adductor brevis (O.)

Gracilis (O.)

Ilio-psoas (I.)

Adductor magnus (O.)

Quadratus femoris (O.)

Obturator externus (O.)

Vastus intermedius (O.)

Articularis genu (O.)

Femur

Quadriceps femoris (I.)

Adductor magnus (I.)

Patella

Attachment of posterior part of
ilio-tibial tract of fascia lata

Vastus lateralis (I.)

Biceps femoris (I.)

Vastus medialis (I.)

Ligamentum patellæ

Peronæus longus (O.)

Gracilis (I.)

Semitendinosus (I.)

Extensor digitorum longus (O.)

Sartorius (I.)

Tibialis anterior (O.)

Fibula

Anterior border of tibia

Peronæus brevis (O.)

Medial border of tibia

Extensor hallucis longus (O.)

Lateral malleolus

Medial malleolus

Extensor digitorum brevis (O.)

Peronæus tertius (O. and I.)

Peronæus brevis (I.)

Tibialis anterior (I.)

4th dorsal interosseous

Extensor digitorum brevis (I.)

Middle slip
and collateral slips of extensor
expansion

Extensor hallucis longus (I.)

3rd dorsal interosseous

2nd dorsal interosseous   1st dorsal interosseous

Glutæus medius (O.)

Glutæus minimus (O.)

Reflected tendon of rectus femoris (O.)

Glutæus maximus (O.)

Gemellus superior (O.)

Gemellus inferior (O.)

Obturator externus (I.)

Obturator internus (O.)

Glutæus medius (I.)

Semimembranosus (O.)

Quadratus femoris (I.)

Biceps femoris (long head) (O.)

Ilio-psoas (I.)

Pectineus (I.)

Semitendinosus (O.)

Glutæus maximus (I.)

Adductor brevis (I.)

Vastus intermedius (O.)

Adductor longus (I.)

Vastus medialis (O.)

Vastus lateralis (O.)

Biceps femoris (short head) (O.)

Adductor magnus (I.)

Plantaris (O.)

Gastrocnemius (medial head) (O.)

Gastrocnemius (lateral head) (O.)

Popliteus (O.)

Femur : medial condyle

Membranous insertion of semimembranosus entering into formation of oblique ligament

Tendinous insertion of semimembranosus

Soleus (O.)

Tibialis posterior (O.)

Popliteus (I.)

Flexor hallucis longus (O.)

Flexor digitorum longus (O.)

Tibia

Peronæus brevis (O.)

Fibula

Attachment of tendo calcaneus and of tendon of plantaris

Abductor digiti minimi (O.)

Flexor digitorum brevis (O.)

Accessory slip of flexor digitorum longus (I.)

Abductor hallucis (O.)

Tibialis posterior (I.)

Flexor digiti minimi brevis (O.)

Tibialis anterior (I.)

Adductor hallucis (O.)

Peronæus longus (I.)

Flexor digitorum brevis and abductor digiti minimi (I.)

Abductor hallucis (I.)

Flexor hallucis brevis (O. and I.)

Adductor hallucis (I.)

3rd plantar interosseous

Flexor hallucis longus (I.)

2nd plantar interosseous

1st plantar interosseous

Flexor digitorum brevis (I.)

Flexor digitorum longus (I.)

PLATE 60.—MANDIBULAR JOINT

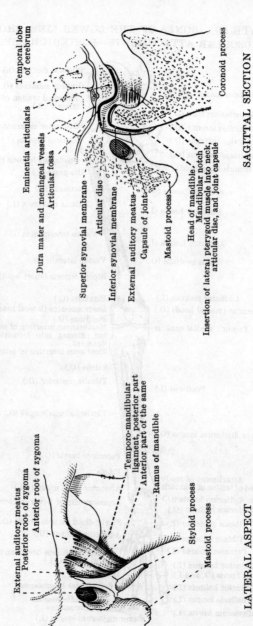

SAGITTAL SECTION

Temporal lobe of cerebrum

Coronoid process

Eminentia articularis

Dura mater and meningeal vessels

Articular fossa

Superior synovial membrane

Articular disc

Inferior synovial membrane

External auditory meatus

Capsule of joint

Mastoid process

Head of mandible

Mandibular notch

Insertion of lateral pterygoid muscle into neck, articular disc, and joint capsule

LATERAL ASPECT

External auditory meatus

Posterior root of zygoma

Anterior root of zygoma

Temporo-mandibular ligament, posterior part

Anterior part of the same

Ramus of mandible

Styloid process

Mastoid process

PLATE 61.—MANDIBULAR JOINT—MEDIAL ASPECT

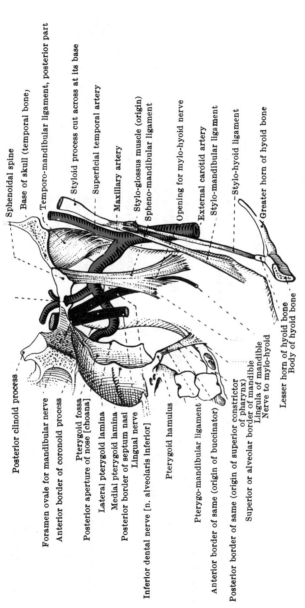

Foramen spinosum for middle meningeal artery, vein, and nervus spinosus

Posterior clinoid process

Sphenoidal spine

Base of skull (temporal bone)

Temporo-mandibular ligament, posterior part

Styloid process cut across at its base

Superficial temporal artery

Foramen ovale for mandibular nerve

Anterior border of coronoid process

Maxillary artery

Stylo-glossus muscle (origin)

Pterygoid fossa

Spheno-mandibular ligament

Posterior aperture of nose [choana]

Lateral pterygoid lamina

Opening for mylo-hyoid nerve

Medial pterygoid lamina

External carotid artery

Posterior border of septum nasi

Stylo-mandibular ligament

Lingual nerve

Stylo-hyoid ligament

Inferior dental nerve [n. alveolaris inferior]

Greater horn of hyoid bone

Pterygoid hamulus

Pterygo-mandibular ligament

Anterior border of same (origin of buccinator)

Posterior border of same (origin of superior constrictor of pharynx)

Lingula of mandible

Superior or alveolar border of mandible

Nerve to mylo-hyoid

Lesser horn of hyoid bone

Body of hyoid bone

PLATE 62.—POSTERIOR LIGAMENTS OF NECK AND SAGITTAL SECTION THROUGH ATLANTO-OCCIPITAL AND ATLANTO-AXIAL JOINTS

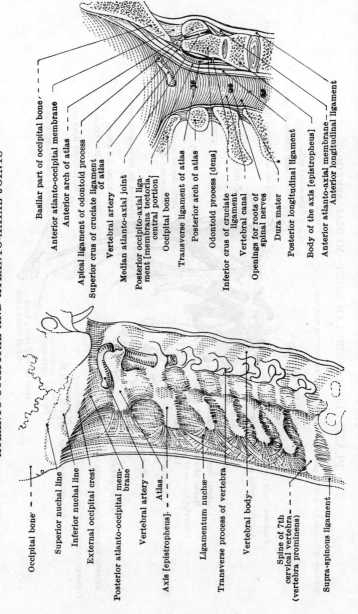

Basilar part of occipital bone

Anterior atlanto-occipital membrane

Anterior arch of atlas

Apical ligament of odontoid process

Superior crus of cruciate ligament of atlas

Vertebral artery

Median atlanto-axial joint

Posterior occipito-axial ligament [membrana tectoria, central portion]

Occipital bone

Transverse ligament of atlas

Posterior arch of atlas

Odontoid process [dens]

Inferior crus of cruciate ligament

Vertebral canal

Openings for roots of spinal nerves

Dura mater

Posterior longitudinal ligament

Body of the axis [epistropheus]

Anterior atlanto-axial membrane

Anterior longitudinal ligament

Occipital bone

Superior nuchal line

Inferior nuchal line

External occipital crest

Posterior atlanto-occipital membrane

Vertebral artery

Atlas

Axis [epistropheus]

Ligamentum nuchae

Transverse process of vertebra

Vertebral body

Spine of 7th cervical vertebra (vertebra prominens)

Supra-spinous ligament

PLATE 63.—COSTO-VERTEBRAL JOINT. HORIZONTAL SECTION AND LEFT LATERAL ASPECT

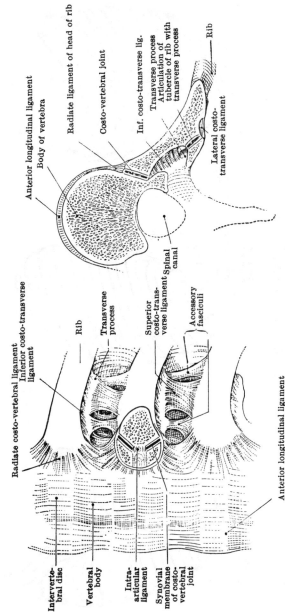

Anterior longitudinal ligament
Body of vertebra
Radiate ligament of head of rib
Costo-vertebral joint
Inf. costo-transverse lig.
Transverse process
Articulation of tubercle of rib with transverse process
Rib
Lateral costo-transverse ligament

Radiate costo-vertebral ligament
Inferior costo-transverse ligament
Rib
Transverse process
Superior costo-transverse ligament
Spinal canal
Accessory fasciculi

Intervertebral disc
Vertebral body
Intra-articular ligament
Synovial membrane of costo-vertebral joint
Anterior longitudinal ligament

PLATE 64.—THE THORACIC CAGE

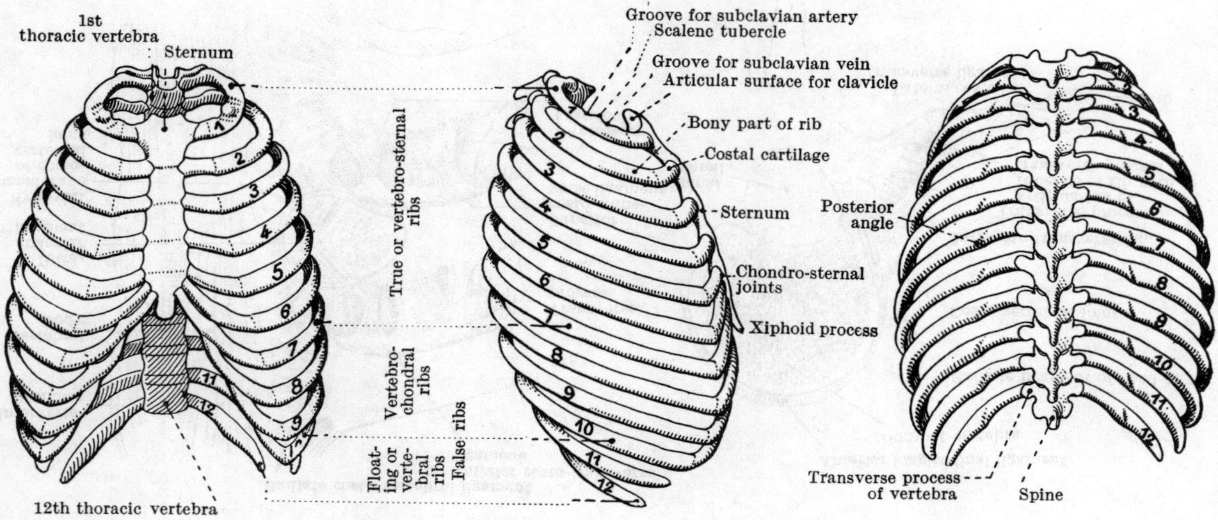

POSTERIOR ASPECT

Spine

Transverse process of vertebra

Groove for subclavian artery
Scalene tubercle

Groove for subclavian vein
Articular surface for clavicle

Bony part of rib

Costal cartilage

Sternum

Posterior angle

Chondro-sternal joints

Xiphoid process

RIGHT LATERAL ASPECT

True or vertebro-sternal ribs

Vertebro-chondral ribs

Floating or vertebral ribs

False ribs

ANTERIOR ASPECT

1st thoracic vertebra

Sternum

12th thoracic vertebra

PLATE 65.—STERNO-COSTO-CLAVICULAR JOINTS

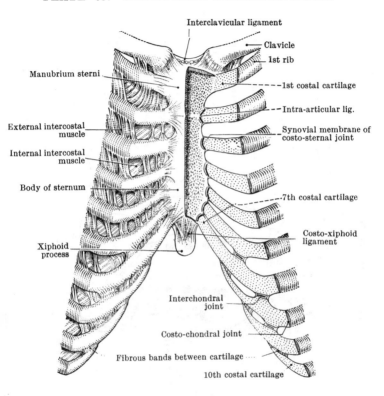

Interclavicular ligament

Clavicle

1st rib

Manubrium sterni

1st costal cartilage

Intra-articular lig.

Synovial membrane of costo-sternal joint

External intercostal muscle

Internal intercostal muscle

Body of sternum

7th costal cartilage

Costo-xiphoid ligament

Xiphoid process

Interchondral joint

Costo-chondral joint

Fibrous bands between cartilage

10th costal cartilage

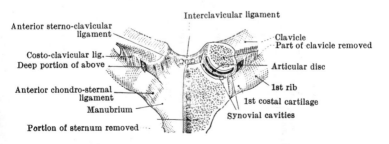

Interclavicular ligament

Anterior sterno-clavicular ligament

Clavicle
Part of clavicle removed

Costo-clavicular lig.
Deep portion of above

Articular disc

Anterior chondro-sternal ligament

1st rib

Manubrium

1st costal cartilage

Synovial cavities

Portion of sternum removed

PLATE 66.—JOINTS OF THE PELVIS

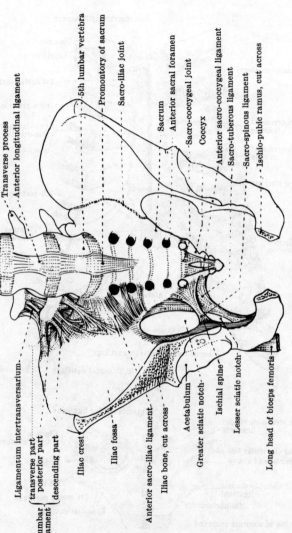

Ligamentum intertransversarium

Ilio-lumbar { transverse part
ligament { posterior part
{ descending part

Transverse process

Anterior longitudinal ligament

5th lumbar vertebra

Promontory of sacrum

Sacro-iliac joint

Iliac crest

Iliac fossa

Anterior sacro-iliac ligament

Iliac bone, cut across

Greater sciatic notch

Acetabulum

Ischial spine

Lesser sciatic notch

Long head of biceps femoris

Sacrum

Anterior sacral foramen

Anterior sacro-coccygeal joint

Coccyx

Anterior sacro-coccygeal ligament

Sacro-tuberous ligament

Sacro-spinous ligament

Ischio-pubic ramus, cut across

ANTERIOR ASPECT

PLATE 67.—JOINTS OF THE PELVIS

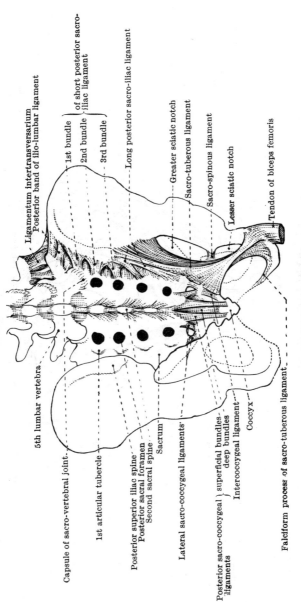

Ligamentum intertransversarium
Posterior band of ilio-lumbar ligament

1st bundle
2nd bundle } of short posterior sacro-iliac ligament
3rd bundle

Long posterior sacro-iliac ligament

Greater sciatic notch

Sacro-tuberous ligament

Sacro-spinous ligament

Lesser sciatic notch

Tendon of biceps femoris

5th lumbar vertebra

Capsule of sacro-vertebral joint

1st articular tubercle

Posterior superior iliac spine
Posterior sacral foramen
Second sacral spine

Sacrum

Lateral sacro-coccygeal ligaments

Posterior sacro-coccygeal } superficial bundles
ligaments } deep bundles

Intercoccygeal ligament

Coccyx

Falciform process of sacro-tuberous ligament

POSTERIOR ASPECT

PLATE 68.—ANTERO-POSTERIOR DIAMETERS OF THE PELVIS

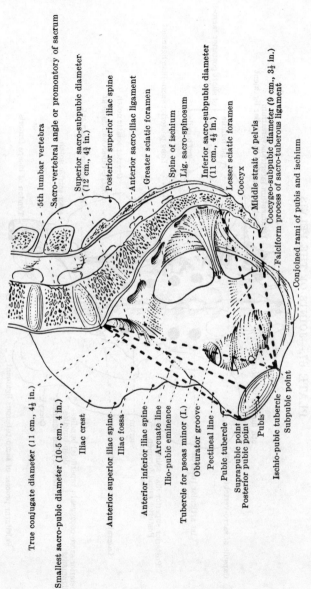

True conjugate diameter (11 cm., 4⅓ in.)

Smallest sacro-pubic diameter (10·5 cm., 4 in.)

Iliac crest

Anterior superior iliac spine

Iliac fossa

Anterior inferior iliac spine

Arcuate line

Ilio-pubic eminence

Tubercle for psoas minor (L.)

Obturator groove

Pectineal line

Pubic tubercle

Suprapubic point

Posterior pubic point

Pubis

Ischio-pubic tubercle

Subpubic point

5th lumbar vertebra

Sacro-vertebral angle or promontory of sacrum

Superior sacro-subpubic diameter (12 cm., 4¾ in.)

Posterior superior iliac spine

Anterior sacro-iliac ligament

Greater sciatic foramen

Spine of ischium

Lig. sacro-spinosum

Inferior sacro-subpubic diameter (11 cm., 4⅓ in.)

Lesser sciatic foramen

Coccyx

Middle strait of pelvis

Coccygeo-subpubic diameter (9 cm., 3½ in.)

Falciform process of sacro-tuberous ligament

Conjoined rami of pubis and ischium

PLATE 69.—DIAGRAMS OF PELVIC OUTLET

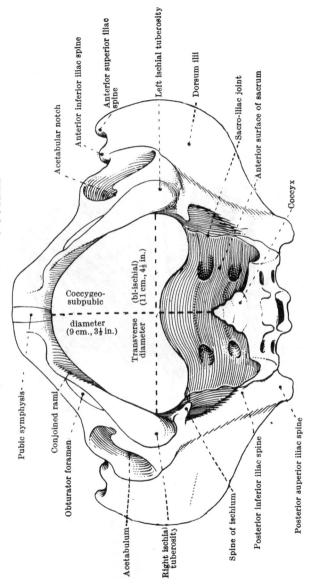

Acetabular notch

Anterior inferior iliac spine

Anterior superior iliac spine

Left ischial tuberosity

Dorsum ilii

Sacro-iliac joint

Anterior surface of sacrum

Coccyx

Pubic symphysis

Conjoined rami

Obturator foramen

Acetabulum

Right ischial tuberosity

Spine of ischium

Posterior inferior iliac spine

Posterior superior iliac spine

Coccygeo-subpubic diameter (9 cm., 3½ in.)

Transverse diameter (bi-ischial, 4⅜ in.) (11 cm.)

PLATE 70.—SHOULDER JOINT

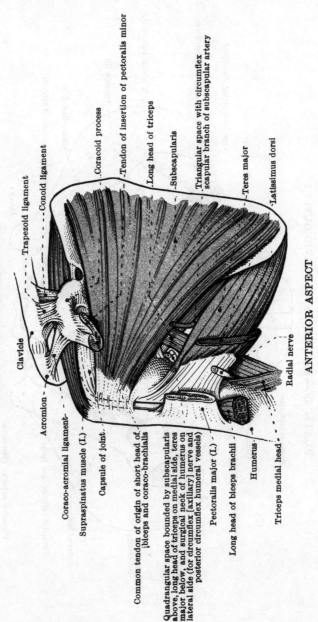

Trapezoid ligament
Conoid ligament
Coracoid process
Tendon of insertion of pectoralis minor
Long head of triceps
Subscapularis
Triangular space with circumflex scapular branch of subscapular artery
Teres major
Latissimus dorsi
Clavicle
Acromion
Coraco-acromial ligament
Supraspinatus muscle (L.)
Capsule of joint
Common tendon of origin of short head of [biceps and coraco-brachialis
Quadrangular space bounded by subscapularis above, long head of triceps on medial side, teres major below, and surgical neck of humerus on lateral side (for circumflex [axillary] nerve and posterior circumflex humeral vessels)
Pectoralis major (L.)
Long head of biceps brachii
Humerus
Triceps medial head
Radial nerve

ANTERIOR ASPECT

PLATE 71.—SHOULDER JOINT

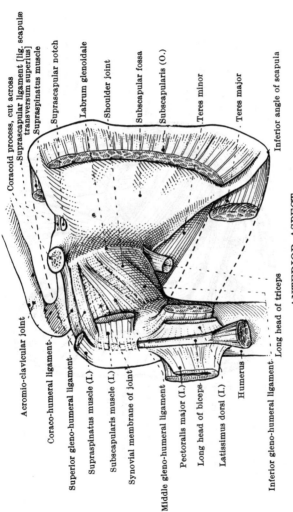

Coracoid process, cut across
Suprascapular ligament [lig. scapulæ transversum superius]
Supraspinatus muscle
Suprascapular notch
Labrum glenoidale
Shoulder joint
Subscapular fossa
Subscapularis (O.)
Teres minor
Teres major
Inferior angle of scapula

Acromio-clavicular joint
Coraco-humeral ligament
Superior gleno-humeral ligament
Supraspinatus muscle (I.)
Subscapularis muscle (I.)
Synovial membrane of joint
Middle gleno-humeral ligament
Pectoralis major (I.)
Long head of biceps
Latissimus dorsi (I.)
Humerus
Long head of triceps
Inferior gleno-humeral ligament

ANTERIOR ASPECT
[DEEPER DISSECTION]

PLATE 72.—SHOULDER JOINT

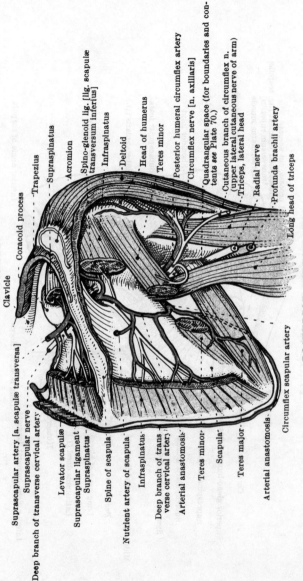

Suprascapular artery [a. scapulæ transversa]
Suprascapular nerve
Deep branch of transverse cervical artery
Levator scapulæ
Suprascapular ligament
Supraspinatus
Spine of scapula
Nutrient artery of scapula
Infraspinatus
Deep branch of trans verse cervical artery
Arterial anastomosis
Teres minor
Scapula
Teres major
Arterial anastomosis
Circumflex scapular artery

Clavicle
Coracoid process
Trapezius
Supraspinatus
Acromion
Spino-glenoid lig. [lig. scapulæ transversum inferius]
Infraspinatus
Deltoid
Head of humerus
Teres minor
Posterior humeral circumflex artery
Quadrangular space [n. axillaris]
Circumflex nerve [n. axillaris]
Cutaneous branch of circumflex n. (upper lateral cutaneous nerve of arm)
Triceps, lateral head
Radial nerve
Profunda brachii artery
Long head of triceps

POSTERIOR ASPECT

PLATE 73.—SHOULDER JOINT

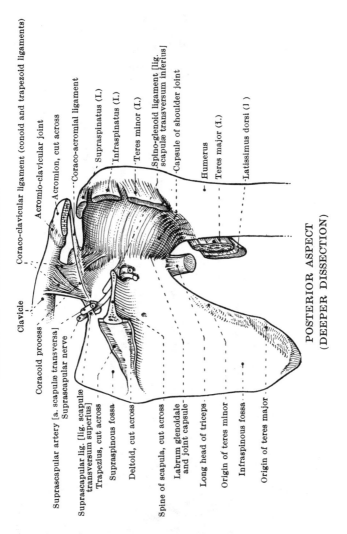

Clavicle

Coracoid process

Coraco-clavicular ligament (conoid and trapezoid ligaments)

Acromio-clavicular joint

Acromion, cut across

Coraco-acromial ligament

Suprascapular artery [a. scapulæ transversa]
Suprascapular nerve

Suprascapular lig. [lig. scapulæ transversum superius]
Trapezius, cut across
Supraspinous fossa

Deltoid, cut across

Spine of scapula, cut across

Labrum glenoidale and joint capsule

Long head of triceps

Origin of teres minor

Infraspinous fossa

Origin of teres major

Supraspinatus (I.)

Infraspinatus (I.)

Teres minor (I.)

Spino-glenoid ligament [lig. scapulæ transversum inferius]

Capsule of shoulder joint

Humerus

Teres major (I.)

Latissimus dorsi (I.)

POSTERIOR ASPECT
(DEEPER DISSECTION)

PLATE 74.—ELBOW JOINT

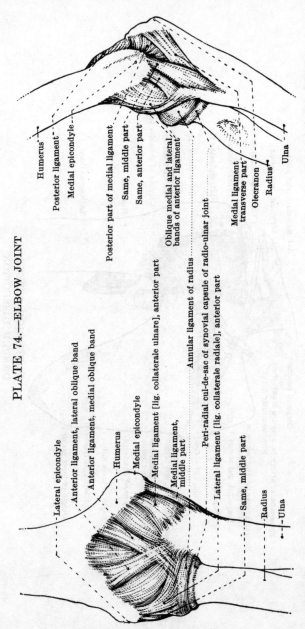

ANTERIOR ASPECT

- - - Lateral epicondyle
- - - Anterior ligament, lateral oblique band
- - - Anterior ligament, medial oblique band
- - - Humerus
- - - Medial epicondyle
- - - Medial ligament [lig. collaterale ulnare], anterior part.
- - - Medial ligament, middle part
- - - Same, middle part
- - - Peri-radial cul-de-sac of synovial capsule of radio-ulnar joint
- - - Lateral ligament [lig. collaterale radiale], anterior part.
- - - Radius
- - - Ulna

MEDIAL ASPECT

- - - Humerus
- - - Posterior ligament
- - - Medial epicondyle
- - - Posterior part of medial ligament
- - - Same, middle part
- - - Same, anterior part
- - - Oblique medial and lateral bands of anterior ligament
- - - Annular ligament of radius
- - - Medial ligament transverse part
- - - Olecranon
- - - Radius
- - - Ulna

PLATE 75.—ELBOW JOINT

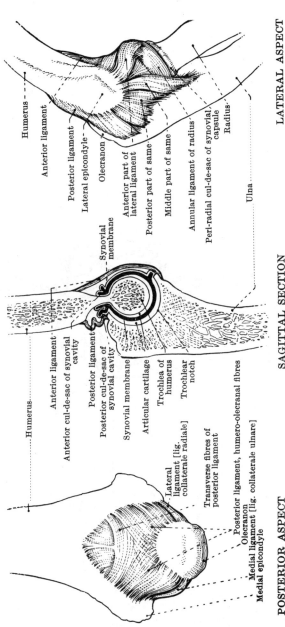

POSTERIOR ASPECT

Humerus

Lateral ligament [lig. collaterale radiale]

Transverse fibres of posterior ligament

Posterior ligament, humero-olecranal fibres
Olecranon
Medial ligament [lig. collaterale ulnare]
Medial epicondyle

SAGITTAL SECTION

Humerus

Anterior ligament

Anterior cul-de-sac of synovial cavity

Posterior ligament
Posterior cul-de-sac of synovial cavity
Synovial membrane
Articular cartilage
Trochlea of humerus
Trochlear notch

Synovial membrane

LATERAL ASPECT

Humerus

Anterior ligament

Posterior ligament
Lateral epicondyle
Olecranon

Anterior part of lateral ligament
Posterior part of same

Middle part of same

Annular ligament of radius
Peri-radial cul-de-sac of synovial capsule
Radius

Ulna

PLATE 76.—WRIST JOINT

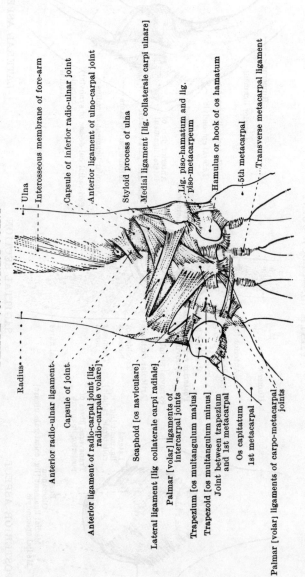

Radius

Anterior radio-ulnar ligament

Capsule of joint

Anterior ligament of radio-carpal joint [lig. radio-carpale volare]

Scaphoid [os naviculare]

Lateral ligament [lig collaterale carpi radiale]

Palmar [volar] ligaments of intercarpal joints

Trapezium [os multangulum majus]

Trapezoid [os multangulum minus]

Joint between trapezium and 1st metacarpal

Os capitatum

1st metacarpal

Palmar [volar] ligaments of carpo-metacarpal joints

Ulna

Interosseous membrane of fore-arm

Capsule of inferior radio-ulnar joint

Anterior ligament of ulno-carpal joint

Styloid process of ulna

Medial ligament [lig. collaterale carpi ulnare]

Lig. piso-hamatum and lig. piso-metacarpeum

Hamulus or hook of os hamatum

5th metacarpal

Transverse metacarpal ligament

PALMAR ASPECT

PLATE 77.—WRIST JOINT

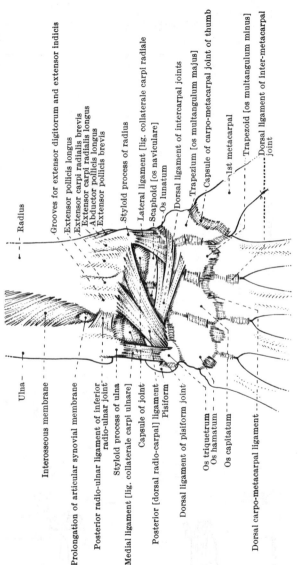

Ulna

Interosseous membrane

Prolongation of articular synovial membrane

Posterior radio-ulnar ligament of inferior radio-ulnar joint

Styloid process of ulna

Medial ligament [lig. collaterale carpi ulnare]

Capsule of joint

Posterior [dorsal radio-carpal] ligament
Pisiform

Dorsal ligament of pisiform joint

Os triquetrum
Os hamatum
Os capitatum

Dorsal carpo-metacarpal ligament

Radius

Grooves for extensor digitorum and extensor indicis

Extensor pollicis longus
Extensor carpi radialis brevis
Extensor carpi radialis longus
Abductor pollicis longus
Extensor pollicis brevis

Styloid process of radius

Lateral ligament [lig. collaterale carpi radiale]
Scaphoid [os naviculare]
Os lunatum

Dorsal ligament of intercarpal joints

Trapezium [os multangulum majus]

Capsule of carpo-metacarpal joint of thumb

1st metacarpal

Trapezoid [os multangulum minus]

Dorsal ligament of inter-metacarpal joint

DORSAL ASPECT

PLATE 78.—RADIO-ULNAR JOINTS

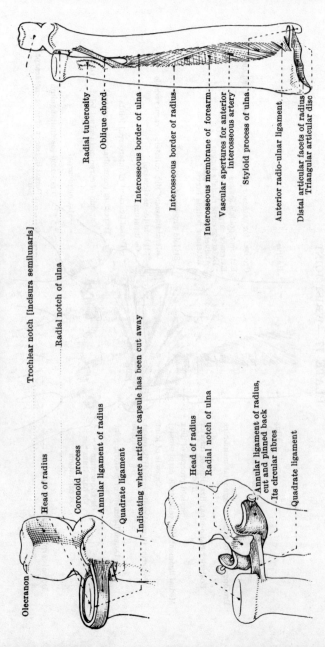

Olecranon

Head of radius

Coronoid process

Annular ligament of radius

Quadrate ligament

Indicating where articular capsule has been cut away

Trochlear notch [incisura semilunaris]

Radial notch of ulna

Head of radius

Radial notch of ulna

Annular ligament of radius, cut and pinned back

Its circular fibres

Quadrate ligament

Radial tuberosity

Oblique chord

Interosseous border of ulna

Interosseous border of radius

Interosseous membrane of forearm

Vascular apertures for anterior interosseous artery

Styloid process of ulna

Anterior radio-ulnar ligament

Distal articular facets of radius

Triangular articular disc

PLATE 78.—JOINTS OF THE FINGERS

Labels (left diagram, reading from top):

Distal phalanx

Tendon of flexor digitorum profundus (perforating, with its vinculum breve)
Tendon of extensor
Collateral ligament
Capsule of joint

Palmar ligament

Middle phalanx

Extensor tendon
Synovial membrane
Collateral ligament
Capsule of joint
Tendon of flexor digitorum sublimis (perforated)

Synovial cleft

Proximal phalanx

Collateral ligament
Capsule of joint
Synovial membrane

Metacarpo-phalangeal joint

Articular fibro-cartilag.

Palmar synovial cul-de-sac

Metacarpo-phalangeal joint

Dorsal synovial cul-de-sac

Metacarpal bone

Labels (center diagram, reading from top):

Synovial cleft
Capsule of joint
Dorsal synovial cul-de-sac
Palmar synovial cul-de-sac

Dorsal synovial cul-de-sac
Capsule of joint
Palmar ligament
Palmar synovial cul-de-sac

Capsule of joint

Interphalangeal joint

Middle phalanx

Interphalangeal joint

Labels (right diagram):

Metacarpo-phalangeal joint

Proximal phalanx

Collateral ligaments
Metacarpal bone

Distal phalanx

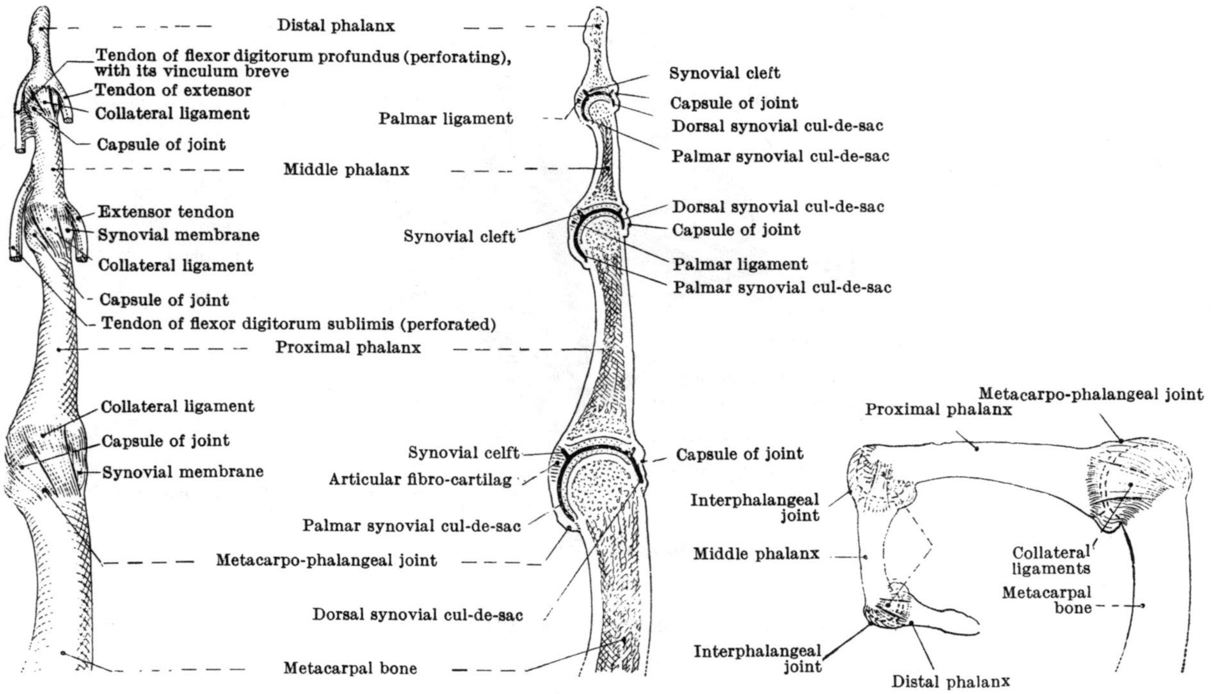

PLATE 80.—HIP JOINT

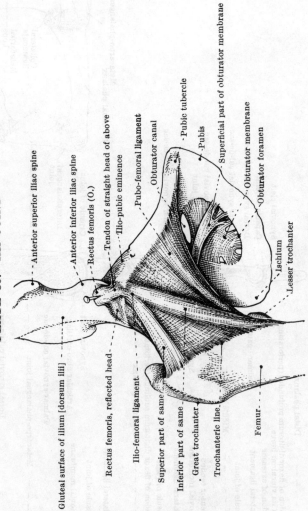

Gluteal surface of ilium [dorsum ilii]

Rectus femoris, reflected head

Ilio-femoral ligament

Superior part of same

Inferior part of same

Great trochanter

Trochanteric line

Femur

Anterior superior iliac spine

Anterior inferior iliac spine

Rectus femoris (O.)

Tendon of straight head of above

Ilio-pubic eminence

Pubo-femoral ligament

Obturator canal

Pubic tubercle

Pubis

Superficial part of obturator membrane

Obturator membrane

Obturator foramen

Ischium

Lesser trochanter

ANTERIOR ASPECT

PLATE 81.—HIP JOINT

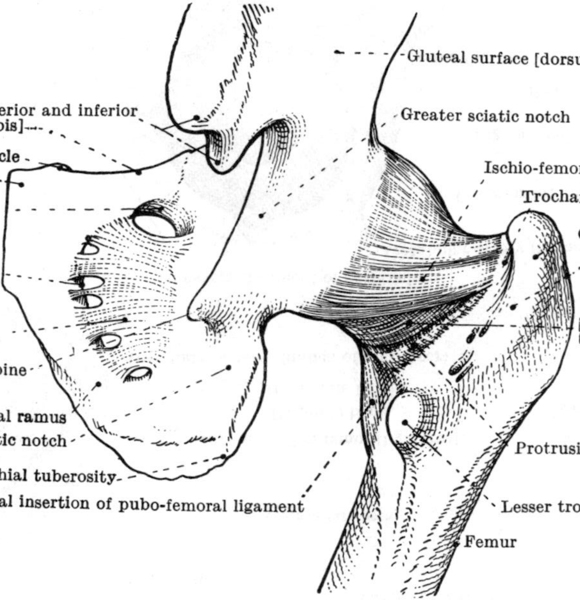

POSTERIOR ASPECT

Gluteal surface [dorsum ilii]

Greater sciatic notch

Ischio-femoral ligament

Trochanteric fossa

Greater trochanter

Trochanteric crest

[Zona orbicularis] (circular fibres of the articular capsule, posterior part)

Protrusion of synovial membrane of joint

Lesser trochanter

Femur

Posterior iliac spines, superior and inferior
Pectineal line [pecten ossis pubis]

Pubic tubercle

Pubis

Obturator canal

Margin of obturator foramen

Obturator membrane

Ischial spine

Ischial ramus

Lesser sciatic notch

Ischial tuberosity

Lower or femoral insertion of pubo-femoral ligament

6

PLATE 82.—DETAILS OF HIP JOINT

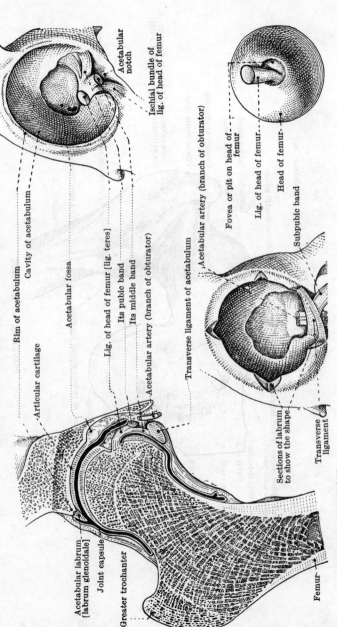

Rim of acetabulum

Cavity of acetabulum

Acetabular fossa

Lig. of head of femur [lig. teres]

Its pubic band

Its middle band

Acetabular artery (branch of obturator)

Transverse ligament of acetabulum

Acetabular labrum [labrum glenoidale]

Joint capsule

Greater trochanter

Femur

VERTICAL SECTION
THROUGH HIP JOINT

Acetabular notch

Ischial bundle of
lig. of head of femur

Articular cartilage

Acetabular artery (branch of obturator)

Fovea or pit on head of femur

Lig. of head of femur

Head of femur

Subpubic band

Sections of labrum
to show the shape

Transverse
ligament

PLATE 83.—HORIZONTAL SECTION OF KNEE

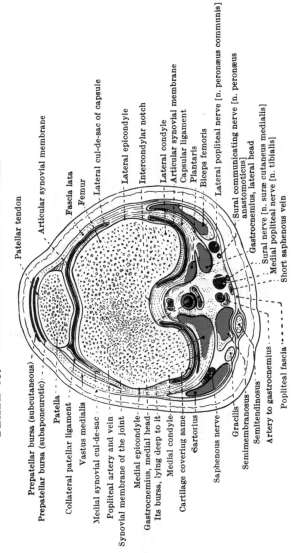

Prepatellar bursa (subcutaneous)
Prepatellar bursa (subaponeurotic)
Patella
Collateral patellar ligament
Vastus medialis
Medial synovial cul-de-sac
Popliteal artery and vein
Synovial membrane of the joint
Medial epicondyle
Gastrocnemius, medial head
Its bursa, lying deep to it
Medial condyle
Cartilage covering same
Sartorius
Saphenous nerve
Gracilis
Semimembranosus
Semitendinosus
Artery to gastrocnemius
Popliteal fascia

Patellar tendon
Articular synovial membrane
Fascia lata
Femur
Lateral cul-de-sac of capsule
Lateral epicondyle
Intercondylar notch
Lateral condyle
Articular synovial membrane
Capsular ligament
Plantaris
Biceps femoris
Lateral popliteal nerve [n. peronæus communis]
Sural communicating nerve [n. peronæus anastomoticus]
Gastrocnemius, lateral head
Sural nerve [n. suræ cutaneus medialis]
Medial popliteal nerve [n. tibialis]
Short saphenous vein

PLATE 84.—KNEE JOINT

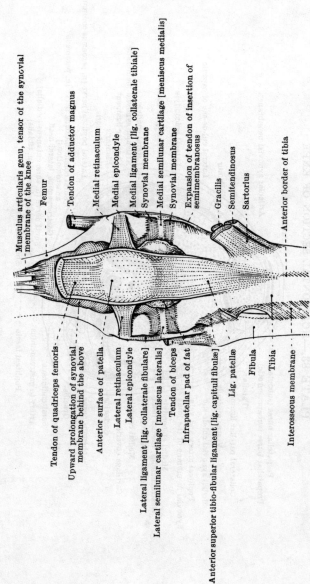

Musculus articularis genu, tensor of the synovial membrane of the knee

Femur

Tendon of adductor magnus

Medial retinaculum

Medial epicondyle

Medial ligament [lig. collaterale tibiale]

Synovial membrane

Medial semilunar cartilage [meniscus medialis]

Synovial membrane

Expansion of tendon of insertion of semimembranosus

Gracilis

Semitendinosus

Sartorius

Anterior border of tibia

Tendon of quadriceps femoris

Upward prolongation of synovial membrane behind the above

Anterior surface of patella

Lateral retinaculum

Lateral epicondyle

Lateral ligament [lig. collaterale fibulare]

Lateral semilunar cartilage [meniscus lateralis]

Tendon of biceps

Infrapatellar pad of fat

Anterior superior tibio-fibular ligament [lig. capituli fibulae]

Lig. patellæ

Fibula

Tibia

Interosseous membrane

ANTERIOR ASPECT

PLATE 85.—KNEE JOINT

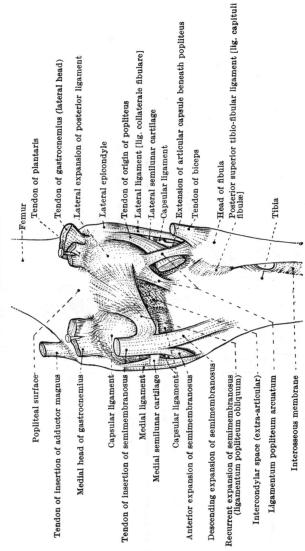

Popliteal surface

Tendon of insertion of adductor magnus

Medial head of gastrocnemius

Capsular ligament

Tendon of insertion of semimembranosus

Medial ligament

Medial semilunar cartilage

Capsular ligament

Anterior expansion of semimembranosus

Descending expansion of semimembranosus

Recurrent expansion of semimembranosus
(ligamentum popliteum obliquum)

Intercondylar space (extra-articular)

Ligamentum popliteum arcuatum

Interosseous membrane

Femur

Tendon of plantaris

Tendon of gastrocnemius (lateral head)

Lateral expansion of posterior ligament

Lateral epicondyle

Tendon of origin of popliteus

Lateral ligament [lig. collaterale fibulare]

Lateral semilunar cartilage

Capsular ligament

Extension of articular capsule beneath popliteus

Tendon of biceps

Head of fibula

Posterior superior tibio-fibular ligament [lig. capituli
fibulæ]

Tibia

POSTERIOR ASPECT

PLATE 86.—KNEE JOINT

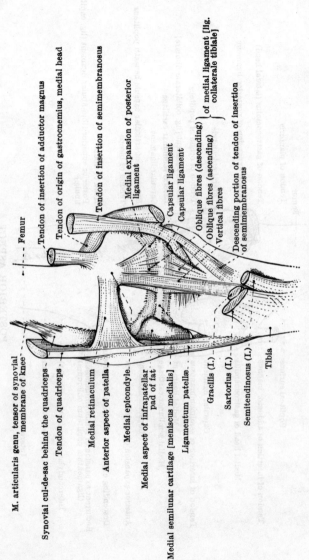

M. articularis genu, tensor of synovial membrane of knee

Synovial cul-de-sac behind the quadriceps

Tendon of quadriceps

Medial retinaculum

Anterior aspect of patella

Medial epicondyle

Medial aspect of infrapatellar pad of fat

Medial semilunar cartilage [meniscus medialis]

Ligamentum patellæ

Gracilis (I.)

Sartorius (I.)

Semitendinosus (I.)

Tibia

Femur

Tendon of insertion of adductor magnus

Tendon of origin of gastrocnemius, medial head

Tendon of insertion of semimembranosus

Medial expansion of posterior ligament

Capsular ligament

Capsular ligament

Oblique fibres (descending)

Oblique fibres (ascending) } of medial ligament [lig. collaterale tibiale]

Vertical fibres

Descending portion of tendon of insertion of semimembranosus

MEDIAL ASPECT

PLATE 87.—KNEE JOINT

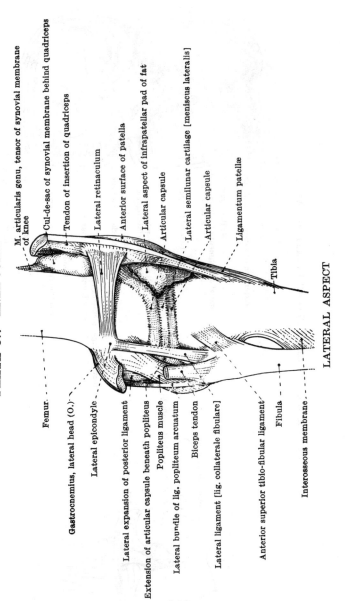

M. articularis genu, tensor of synovial membrane of knee

Cul-de-sac of synovial membrane behind quadriceps

Tendon of insertion of quadriceps

Lateral retinaculum

Anterior surface of patella

Lateral aspect of infrapatellar pad of fat

Articular capsule

Lateral semilunar cartilage [meniscus lateralis]

Articular capsule

Ligamentum patellae

Tibia

Femur

Gastrocnemius, lateral head (O.)

Lateral epicondyle

Lateral expansion of posterior ligament

Extension of articular capsule beneath popliteus

Popliteus muscle

Lateral bundle of lig. popliteum arcuatum

Biceps tendon

Lateral ligament [lig. collaterale fibulare]

Anterior superior tibio-fibular ligament

Fibula

Interosseous membrane

LATERAL ASPECT

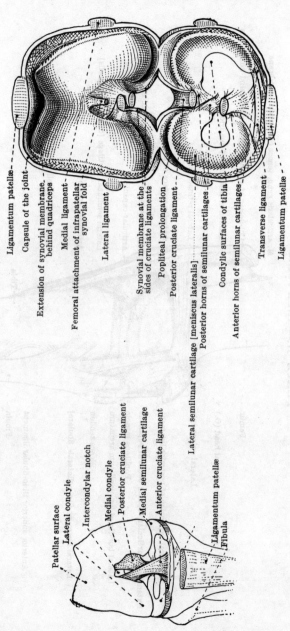

PLATE 88.—KNEE JOINT—CRUCIATE LIGAMENTS

Ligamentum patellae

Capsule of the joint

Extension of synovial membrane, behind quadriceps

Medial ligament

Femoral attachment of infrapatellar synovial fold

Lateral ligament

Synovial membrane at the sides of cruciate ligaments

Popliteal prolongation

Posterior cruciate ligament

Condylic surfaces of tibia

Anterior horns of semilunar cartilages

Transverse ligament

Ligamentum patellae

Lateral semilunar cartilage [meniscus lateralis]

Posterior horns of semilunar cartilages

Patellar surface

Lateral condyle

Intercondylar notch

Medial condyle

Posterior cruciate ligament

Medial semilunar cartilage

Anterior cruciate ligament

Ligamentum patellae

Fibula

PLATE 89.—HORIZONTAL SECTION OF KNEE

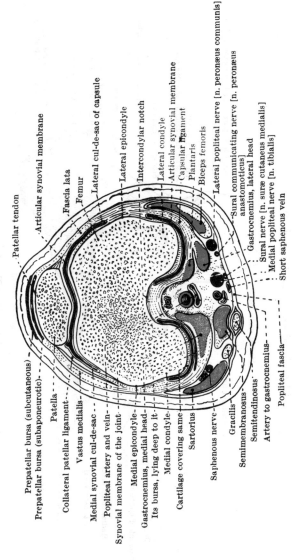

Prepatellar bursa (subcutaneous)
Prepatellar bursa (subaponeurotic)
Patella
Collateral patellar ligament
Vastus medialis
Medial synovial cul-de-sac
Popliteal artery and vein
Synovial membrane of the joint
Medial epicondyle
Gastrocnemius, medial head
Its bursa, lying deep to it
Medial condyle
Cartilage covering same
Sartorius
Saphenous nerve
Gracilis
Semimembranosus
Semitendinosus
Artery to gastrocnemius
Popliteal fascia

Patellar tendon
Articular synovial membrane
Fascia lata
Femur
Lateral cul-de-sac of capsule
Lateral epicondyle
Intercondylar notch
Lateral condyle
Articular synovial membrane
Capsular ligament
Plantaris
Biceps femoris
Lateral popliteal nerve [n. peronæus communis]
Sural communicating nerve [n. peronæus anastomoticus]
Gastrocnemius, lateral head
Sural nerve [n. suræ cutaneus medialis]
Medial popliteal nerve [n. tibialis]
Short saphenous vein

PLATE 90.—JOINTS OF THE FOOT

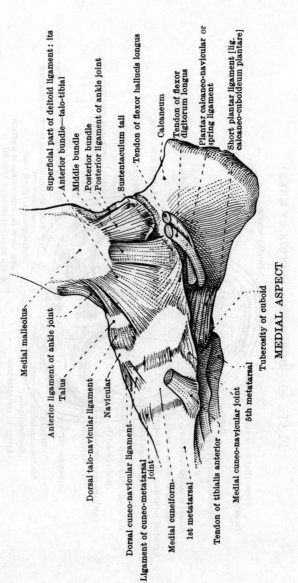

Medial malleolus

Anterior ligament of ankle joint

Talus

Dorsal talo-navicular ligament

Navicular

Dorsal cuneo-navicular ligament

Ligament of cuneo-metatarsal joint

Medial cuneiform

1st metatarsal

Tendon of tibialis anterior

Medial cuneo-navicular joint

5th metatarsal

Tuberosity of cuboid

Superficial part of deltoid ligament: its
Anterior bundle—talo-tibial
Middle bundle
Posterior bundle
Posterior ligament of ankle joint
Sustentaculum tali
Tendon of flexor hallucis longus

Calcaneum

Tendon of flexor
digitorum longus

Plantar calcaneo-navicular or
spring ligament

Short plantar ligament [lig.
calcaneo-cuboideum plantare]

MEDIAL ASPECT

PLATE 91.—JOINTS OF THE FOOT

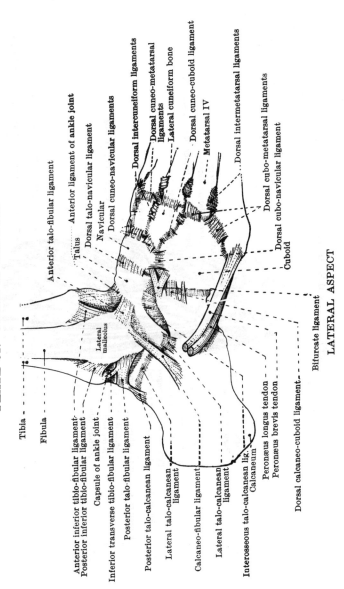

Tibia

Fibula

Anterior inferior tibio-fibular ligament
Posterior inferior tibio-fibular ligament

Capsule of ankle joint

Inferior transverse tibio-fibular ligament

Posterior talo-fibular ligament

Posterior talo-calcanean ligament

Lateral talo-calcanean ligament

Calcaneo-fibular ligament

Lateral talo-calcanean ligament

Interosseous talo-calcanean lig.

Peronaeus longus tendon
Peronaeus brevis tendon

Dorsal calcaneo-cuboid ligament

Anterior talo-fibular ligament

Anterior ligament of ankle joint

Talus

Dorsal talo-navicular ligament

Navicular

Dorsal cuneo-navicular ligaments

Dorsal intercuneiform ligaments

Dorsal cuneo-metatarsal ligaments

Lateral cuneiform bone

Dorsal cuneo-cuboid ligament

Metatarsal IV

Dorsal intermetatarsal ligaments

Dorsal cubo-metatarsal ligaments

Dorsal cubo-navicular ligament

Cuboid

Lateral malleolus

Calcaneum

Bifurcate ligament

LATERAL ASPECT

PLATE 92.—SOLE OF FOOT

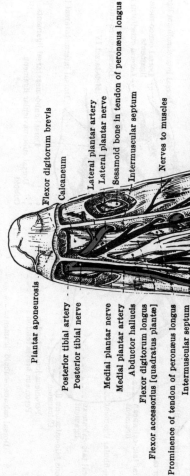

Plantar aponeurosis

Flexor digitorum brevis

Posterior tibial artery
Posterior tibial nerve

Calcaneum

Lateral plantar artery
Lateral plantar nerve
Sesamoid bone in tendon of peronæus longus
Intermuscular septum

Medial plantar nerve
Medial plantar artery
Abductor hallucis
Flexor digitorum longus
Flexor accessorius [quadratus plantæ]

Nerves to muscles

Flexor digiti minimi brevis

Prominence of tendon of peronæus longus
Intermuscular septum
Flexor hallucis longus
Flexor hallucis brevis
1st lumbrical

Deep branch of lateral plantar nerve

Digital arteries and nerves
Plantar aponeurosis (deep fascia)

Tendons, perforated, of flexor digitorum brevis

Tendons, perforating, of flexor digitorum longus]

PLATE 93.—JOINTS OF THE FOOT

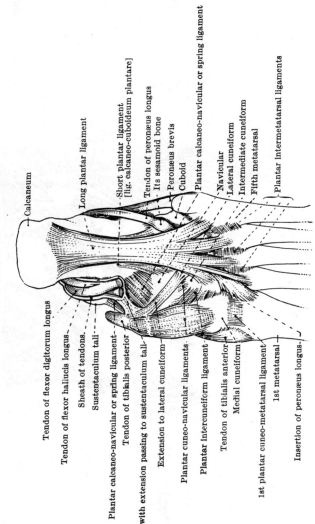

Calcaneum

Tendon of flexor digitorum longus

Tendon of flexor hallucis longus

Sheath of tendons

Sustentaculum tali

Plantar calcaneo-navicular or spring ligament

Tendon of tibialis posterior

with extension passing to sustentaculum tali

Extension to lateral cuneiform

Plantar cuneo-navicular ligaments

Plantar intercuneiform ligament

Tendon of tibialis anterior

Medial cuneiform

1st plantar cuneo-metatarsal ligament

1st metatarsal

Insertion of peroneus longus

Long plantar ligament

Short plantar ligament
[lig. calcaneo-cuboideum plantare]

Tendon of peronaeus longus

Its sesamoid bone

Peronaeus brevis

Cuboid

Plantar calcaneo-navicular or spring ligament

Navicular

Lateral cuneiform

Intermediate cuneiform

Fifth metatarsal

Plantar intermetatarsal ligaments

PLANTAR ASPECT

PLATE 94.—SUPERFICIAL MUSCLES OF SCALP AND FACE

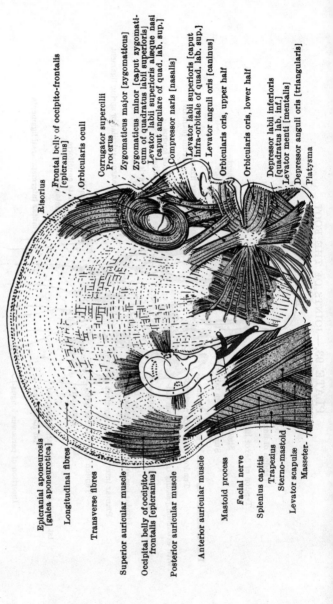

Epicranial aponeurosis [galea aponeurotica]

Longitudinal fibres

Transverse fibres

Superior auricular muscle

Occipital belly of occipito-frontalis [epicranius]

Posterior auricular muscle

Anterior auricular muscle

Mastoid process

Facial nerve

Splenius capitis

Trapezius

Sterno-mastoid

Levator scapulae

Masseter.

Risorius

Frontal belly of occipito-frontalis [epicranius]

Orbicularis oculi

Corrugator supercilii
Procerus

Zygomaticus major [zygomaticus]

Zygomaticus minor [caput zygomaticum of quadratus labii superioris]
Levator labii superioris alaeque nasi [caput angulare of quad. lab. sup.]

Compressor naris [nasalis]

Levator labii superioris [caput infra-orbitale of quad. lab. sup.]

Levator anguli oris [caninus]

Orbicularis oris, upper half

Orbicularis oris, lower half

Depressor labii inferioris [quadratus lab. inf.]
Levator menti [mentalis]

Depressor anguli oris [triangularis]

Platysma

PLATE 95.—SUPERFICIAL MUSCLES OF NECK

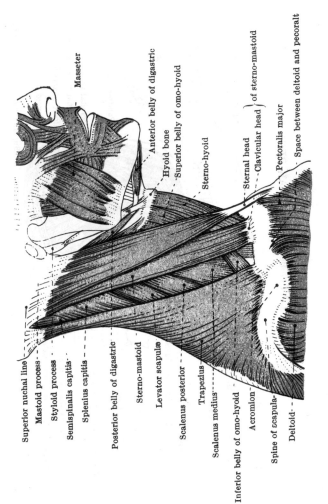

Superior nuchal line
Mastoid process
Styloid process
Semispinalis capitis
Splenius capitis

Posterior belly of digastric
Sterno-mastoid
Levator scapulæ
Scalenus posterior
Trapezius
Scalenus medius
Inferior belly of omo-hyoid
Acromion
Spine of scapula
Deltoid

Masseter

Anterior belly of digastric
Hyoid bone
Superior belly of omo-hyoid

Sterno-hyoid

Sternal head
Clavicular head } of sterno-mastoid

Pectoralis major

Space between deltoid and pecoral†

PLATE 96.—TONSILLAR REGION

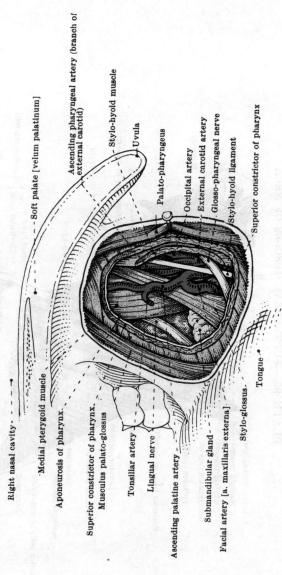

Right nasal cavity

Medial pterygoid muscle

Aponeurosis of pharynx

Superior constrictor of pharynx

Musculus palato-glossus

Tonsillar artery

Lingual nerve

Ascending palatine artery

Submandibular gland

Facial artery [a. maxillaris externa]

Stylo-glossus

Tongue

Soft palate [velum palatinum]

Ascending pharyngeal artery (branch of external carotid)

Stylo-hyoid muscle

Uvula

Palato-pharyngeus

Occipital artery

External carotid artery

Glosso-pharyngeal nerve

Stylo-hyoid ligament

Superior constrictor of pharynx

PLATE 97.—HORIZONTAL SECTION AT LEVEL OF TONSILS

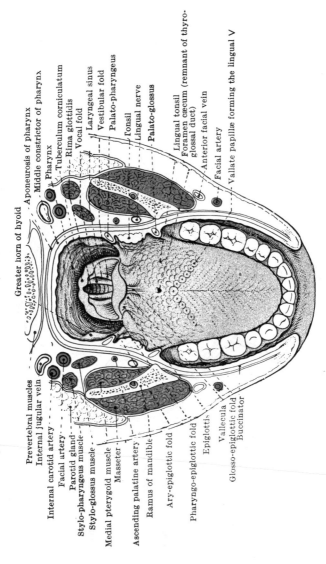

Greater horn of hyoid
Aponeurosis of pharynx
Middle constrictor of pharynx
Pharynx
Tuberculum corniculatum
Rima glottidis
Vocal fold
Laryngeal sinus
Vestibular fold
Palato-pharyngeus
Tonsil
Lingual nerve
Palato-glossus
Lingual tonsil
Foramen caecum (remnant of thyro-glossal duct)
Anterior facial vein
Facial artery
Vallate papillae forming the lingual V

Prevertebral muscles
Internal jugular vein
Internal carotid artery
Facial artery
Parotid gland
Stylo-pharyngeus muscle
Stylo-glossus muscle
Medial pterygoid muscle
Masseter
Ascending palatine artery
Ramus of mandible
Ary-epiglottic fold
Pharyngo-epiglottic fold
Epiglottis
Vallecula
Glosso-epiglottic fold
Buccinator

PLATE 98.—HORIZONTAL SECTION OF EYEBALL [BULBUS OCULI. AND OF OPTIC NERVE

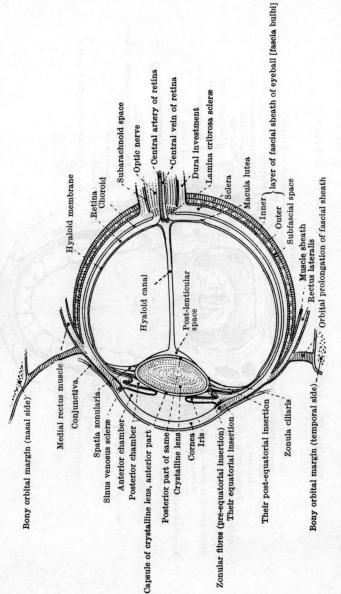

Bony orbital margin (nasal side)

Medial rectus muscle

Conjunctiva

Spatia zonularia

Sinus venosus sclerae

Anterior chamber

Posterior chamber

Capsule of crystalline lens, anterior part

Posterior part of same

Crystalline lens

Cornea

Iris

Zonular fibres (pre-equatorial insertion)
Their equatorial insertion

Their post-equatorial insertion

Zonula ciliaris

Bony orbital margin (temporal side)

Hyaloid membrane

Retina

Choroid

Hyaloid canal

Post-lenticular space

Subarachnoid space

Optic nerve

Central artery of retina

Central vein of retina

Dural investment

Lamina cribrosa sclerae

Sclera

Macula lutea

Inner } layer of fascial sheath of eyeball [fascia bulbi]
Outer }

Subfascial space

Muscle sheath

Rectus lateralis

Orbital prolongation of fascial sheath

PLATE 99.—LACRIMAL APPARATUS

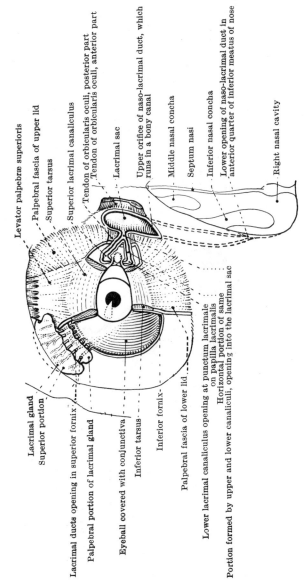

Levator palpebræ superioris

Palpebral fascia of upper lid

Superior tarsus

Superior lacrimal canaliculus

Tendon of orbicularis oculi, posterior part
Tendon of orbicularis oculi, anterior part

Lacrimal sac

Upper orifice of naso-lacrimal duct, which runs in a bony canal

Middle nasal concha

Septum nasi

Inferior nasal concha

Lower opening of naso-lacrimal duct in anterior quarter of inferior meatus of nose

Right nasal cavity

Lacrimal gland
Superior portion

Lacrimal ducts opening in superior fornix

Palpebral portion of lacrimal gland

Eyeball covered with conjunctiva

Inferior tarsus

Inferior fornix

Palpebral fascia of lower lid

Lower lacrimal canaliculus opening at punctum lacrimale on papilla lacrimalis
Horizontal portion of same
Portion formed by upper and lower canaliculi, opening into the lacrimal sac

PLATE 100.—RIGHT ORBIT

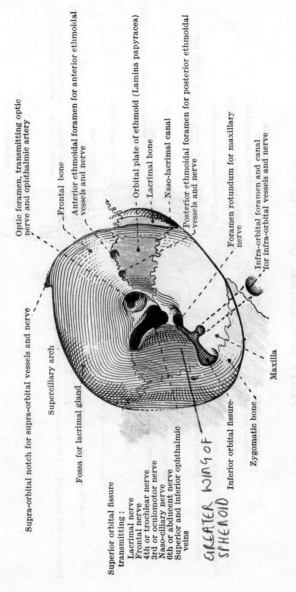

Optic foramen, transmitting optic nerve and ophthalmic artery

Frontal bone

Anterior ethmoidal foramen for anterior ethmoidal vessels and nerve

Orbital plate of ethmoid (Lamina papyracea)

Lacrimal bone

Naso-lacrimal canal

Posterior ethmoidal foramen for posterior ethmoidal vessels and nerve

Foramen rotundum for maxillary nerve

Infra-orbital foramen and canal for infra-orbital vessels and nerve

Maxilla

Supra-orbital notch for supra-orbital vessels and nerve

Superciliary arch

Fossa for lacrimal gland

Superior orbital fissure transmitting :
Lacrimal nerve
Frontal nerve
4th or trochlear nerve
3rd or oculomotor nerve
Naso-ciliary nerve
6th or abducent nerve
Superior and inferior ophthalmic veins

GREATER WING OF SPHENOID

Inferior orbital fissure.

Zygomatic bone

PLATE 101.—RIGHT ORBIT AND THE RELATIONS OF NERVES

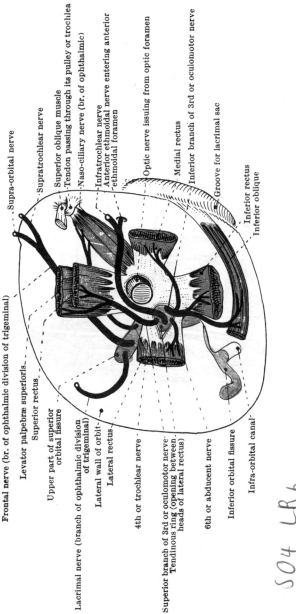

Frontal nerve (br. of ophthalmic division of trigeminal)

Supra-orbital nerve

Supratrochlear nerve

Superior oblique muscle
Tendon passing through its pulley or trochlea

Naso-ciliary nerve (br. of ophthalmic)

Infratrochlear nerve
Anterior ethmoidal nerve entering anterior ethmoidal foramen

Optic nerve issuing from optic foramen

Medial rectus

Inferior branch of 3rd or oculomotor nerve

Groove for lacrimal sac

Inferior rectus
Inferior oblique

Levator palpebræ superioris
Superior rectus

Lacrimal nerve (branch of ophthalmic division of trigeminal)

Upper part of superior orbital fissure

Lateral wall of orbit
Lateral rectus

4th or trochlear nerve

Superior branch of 3rd or oculomotor nerve
Tendinous ring (opening between heads of lateral rectus)

6th or abducent nerve

Inferior orbital fissure

Infra-orbital canal

PLATE 102.—MUSCLES OF THE RIGHT ORBIT—SEEN FROM ABOVE

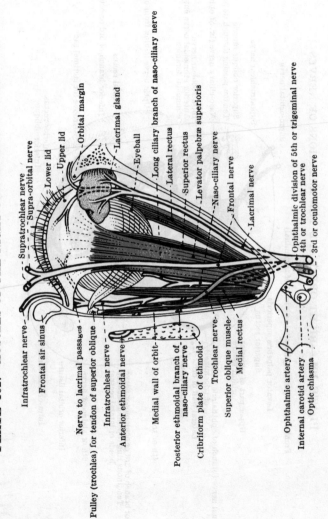

Infratrochlear nerve
Frontal air sinus
Nerve to lacrimal passages
Pulley (trochlea) for tendon of superior oblique
Infratrochlear nerve
Anterior ethmoidal nerve
Medial wall of orbit
Posterior ethmoidal branch of naso-ciliary nerve
Cribriform plate of ethmoid
Trochlear nerve
Superior oblique muscle
Medial rectus
Ophthalmic artery
Internal carotid artery
Optic chiasma

Supratrochlear nerve
Supra-orbital nerve
Lower lid
Upper lid
Orbital margin
Lacrimal gland
Eyeball
Long ciliary branch of naso-ciliary nerve
Lateral rectus
Superior rectus
Levator palpebræ superioris
Naso-ciliary nerve
Frontal nerve
Lacrimal nerve
Ophthalmic division of 5th or trigeminal nerve
4th or trochlear nerve
3rd or oculomotor nerve

PLATE 103.—MUSCLES OF THE RIGHT ORBIT—LATERAL ASPECT

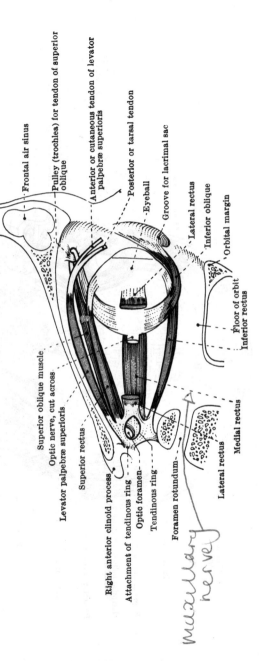

Frontal air sinus

Pulley (trochlea) for tendon of superior oblique

Anterior or cutaneous tendon of levator palpebræ superioris

Posterior or tarsal tendon

Eyeball

Groove for lacrimal sac

Lateral rectus

Inferior oblique

Orbital margin

Floor of orbit

Inferior rectus

Medial rectus

Lateral rectus

Foramen rotundum

Tendinous ring

Optic foramen

Attachment of tendinous ring

Right anterior clinoid process

Superior rectus

Levator palpebræ superioris

Optic nerve, cut across

Superior oblique muscle

Maxillary nerve

PLATE 104.—SUPERFICIAL MUSCLES OF SCALP AND FACE

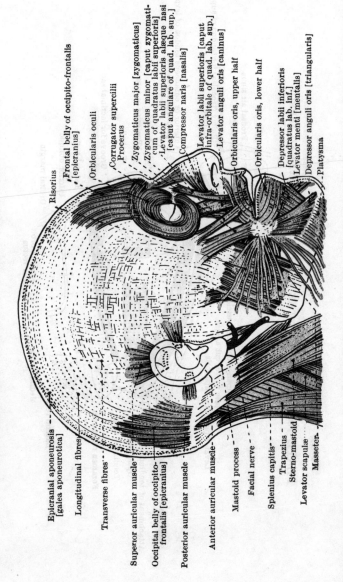

Risorius

Frontal belly of occipito-frontalis [epicranius]

Orbicularis oculi

Corrugator supercilii
Procerus

Zygomaticus major [zygomaticus]

Zygomaticus minor [caput zygomaticum of quadratus labii superioris]
Levator labii superioris alaeque nasi [caput angulare of quad. lab. sup.]

Compressor naris [nasalis]

Levator labii superioris [caput infra-orbitale of quad. lab. sup.]

Levator anguli oris [caninus]

Orbicularis oris, upper half

Orbicularis oris, lower half

Depressor labii inferioris [quadratus lab. inf.]
Levator menti [mentalis]
Depressor anguli oris [triangularis]

Platysma

Epicranial aponeurosis [galea aponeurotica]

Longitudinal fibres

Transverse fibres

Superior auricular muscle

Occipital belly of occipito-frontalis [epicranius]

Posterior auricular muscle

Anterior auricular muscle

Mastoid process

Facial nerve

Splenius capitis
Trapezius
Sterno-mastoid
Levator scapula
Masseter

PLATE 105.—MUSCLES OF NECK (STERNO-MASTOID AND LEVATOR SCAPULÆ HAVE BEEN REMOVED)

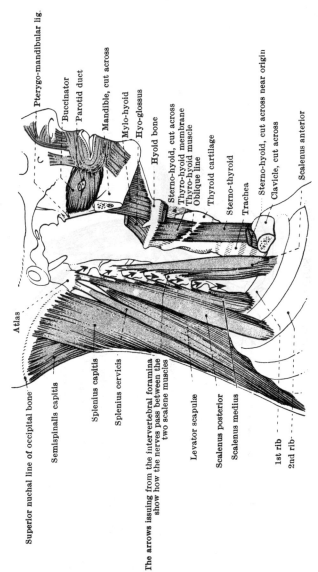

Pterygo-mandibular lig.

Buccinator

Parotid duct

Mandible, cut across

Mylo-hyoid

Hyo-glossus

Hyoid bone

Sterno-hyoid, cut across

Thyro-hyoid membrane

Thyro-hyoid muscle

Oblique line

Thyroid cartilage

Sterno-thyroid

Trachea

Sterno-hyoid, cut across near origin

Clavicle, cut across

Scalenus anterior

Atlas

Superior nuchal line of occipital bone

Semispinalis capitis

Splenius capitis

Splenius cervicis

The **arrows** issuing from the intervertebral foramina show how the nerves pass between the two scalene muscles

Levator scapulæ

Scalenus posterior

Scalenus medius

1st rib

2nd rib

PLATE 106.—MUSCLES OF NECK (*Continued*)

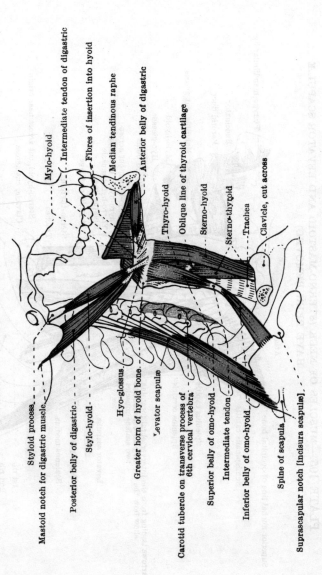

Styloid process

Mastoid notch for digastric muscle

Posterior belly of digastric

Stylo-hyoid

Hyo-glossus

Greater horn of hyoid bone

Carotid tubercle on transverse process of 6th cervical vertebra

Superior belly of omo-hyoid

Intermediate tendon

Inferior belly of omo-hyoid

Spine of scapula

Suprascapular notch [incisura scapulae]

Mylo-hyoid

Intermediate tendon of digastric

Fibres of insertion into hyoid

Median tendinous raphe

Anterior belly of digastric

Thyro-hyoid

Oblique line of thyroid cartilage

Sterno-hyoid

Sterno-thyroid

Trachea

Clavicle, cut across

Levator scapulae

PLATE 107.—MUSCLES OF NECK (Continued)

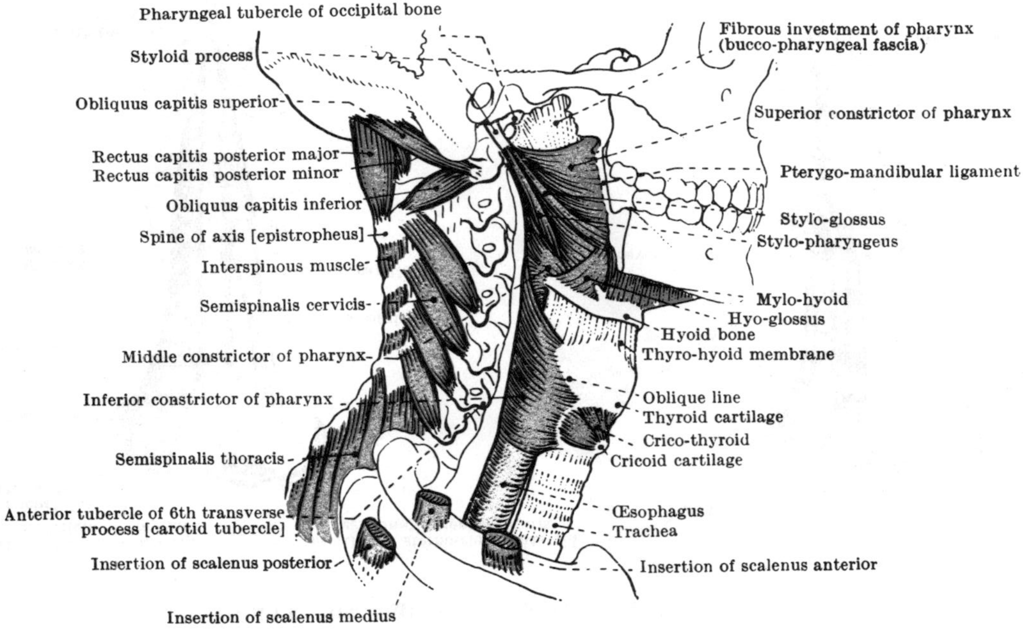

Pharyngeal tubercle of occipital bone

Styloid process

Obliquus capitis superior

Rectus capitis posterior major
Rectus capitis posterior minor

Obliquus capitis inferior

Spine of axis [epistropheus]

Interspinous muscle

Semispinalis cervicis

Middle constrictor of pharynx

Inferior constrictor of pharynx

Semispinalis thoracis

Anterior tubercle of 6th transverse process [carotid tubercle]

Insertion of scalenus posterior

Insertion of scalenus medius

Fibrous investment of pharynx (bucco-pharyngeal fascia)

Superior constrictor of pharynx

Pterygo-mandibular ligament

Stylo-glossus

Stylo-pharyngeus

Mylo-hyoid

Hyo-glossus

Hyoid bone

Thyro-hyoid membrane

Oblique line

Thyroid cartilage

Crico-thyroid

Cricoid cartilage

Œsophagus

Trachea

Insertion of scalenus anterior

PLATE 108.—MUSCLES OF THE BACK OF THE NECK

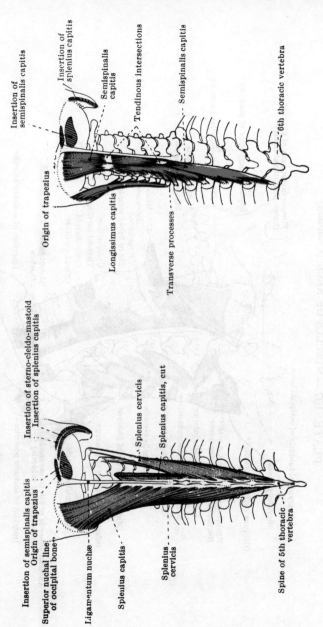

Insertion of semispinalis capitis
Insertion of semispinalis capitis
Insertion of splenius capitis
Semispinalis capitis
Tendinous intersections
Semispinalis capitis
6th thoracic vertebra
Origin of trapezius
Longissimus capitis
Transverse processes

Insertion of semispinalis capitis
Origin of trapezius
Insertion of sterno-cleido-mastoid
Insertion of splenius capitis
Superior nuchal line of occipital bone
Splenius cervicis
Splenius capitis, cut
Ligamentum nuchae
Splenius capitis
Splenius cervicis
Spine of 6th thoracic vertebra

PLATE 109.—PREVERTEBRAL AND SCALENE MUSCLES OF THE NECK

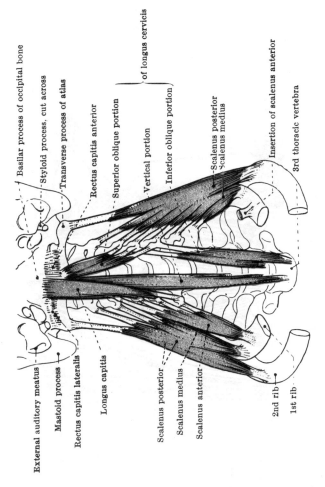

External auditory meatus

Mastoid process

Rectus capitis lateralis

Longus capitis

Scalenus posterior

Scalenus medius

Scalenus anterior

2nd rib

1st rib

Basilar process of occipital bone

Styloid process, cut across

Transverse process of atlas

Rectus capitis anterior

Superior oblique portion

Vertical portion — of longus cervicis

Inferior oblique portion

Scalenus posterior
Scalenus medius

Insertion of scalenus anterior

3rd thoracic vertebra

PLATE 110.—MUSCLES OF THE NECK (ANTERIOR ASPECT)

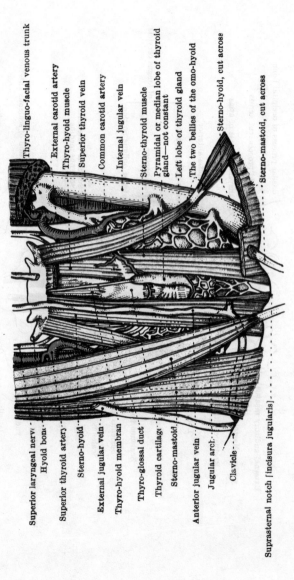

Thyro-linguo-facial venous trunk

External carotid artery

Thyro-hyoid muscle

Superior thyroid vein

Common carotid artery

Internal jugular vein

Sterno-thyroid muscle

Pyramidal or median lobe of thyroid gland—not constant

Left lobe of thyroid gland

The two bellies of the omo-hyoid

Sterno-hyoid, cut across

Sterno-mastoid, cut across

Superior laryngeal nerv·
Hyoid bon·

Superior thyroid artery·
Sterno-hyoid·

External jugular vein·
Thyro-hyoid membran·

Thyro-glossal duct·

Thyroid cartilag·
Sterno-mastoid·

Anterior jugular vein·
Jugular arch·

Clavicle·

Suprasternal notch [Incisura jugularis]·

PLATE 111.—THYROID GLAND AND ITS VESSELS

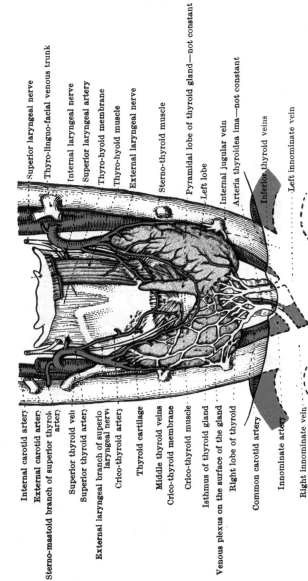

Internal carotid artery
External carotid artery
Sterno-mastoid branch of superior thyroid artery
Superior thyroid vein
Superior thyroid artery
External laryngeal branch of superior laryngeal nerve
Crico-thyroid artery

Thyroid cartilage

Middle thyroid veins
Crico-thyroid membrane

Crico-thyroid muscle
Isthmus of thyroid gland
Venous plexus on the surface of the gland
Right lobe of thyroid

Common carotid artery

Innominate artery

Right innominate vein

Superior laryngeal nerve
Thyro-linguo-facial venous trunk
Internal laryngeal nerve
Superior laryngeal artery
Thyro-hyoid membrane
Thyro-hyoid muscle
External laryngeal nerve

Sterno-thyroid muscle

Pyramidal lobe of thyroid gland—not constant
Left lobe
Internal jugular vein
Arteria thyroidea ima—not constant

Inferior thyroid veins

Left innominate vein

PLATE 112.—COMMON CAROTID ARTERIES

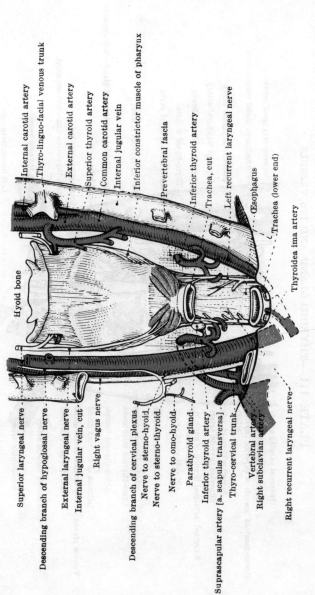

Superior laryngeal nerve

Descending branch of hypoglossal nerve

External laryngeal nerve

Internal jugular vein, cut

Right vagus nerve

Descending branch of cervical plexus

Nerve to sterno-hyoid.

Nerve to sterno-thyroid.

Nerve to omo-hyoid.

Parathyroid gland.

Inferior thyroid artery

Suprascapular artery [a. scapula transversa].

Thyro-cervical trunk

Vertebral artery

Right subclavian artery

Right recurrent laryngeal nerve

Hyoid bone

Internal carotid artery

Thyro-linguo-facial venous trunk

External carotid artery

Superior thyroid artery

Common carotid artery

Internal jugular vein

Inferior constrictor muscle of pharynx

Prevertebral fascia

Inferior thyroid artery

Trachea, cut

Left recurrent laryngeal nerve

Œsophagus

Trachea (lower end)

Thyroidea ima artery

PLATE 113.—TRANSVERSE SECTION OF NECK

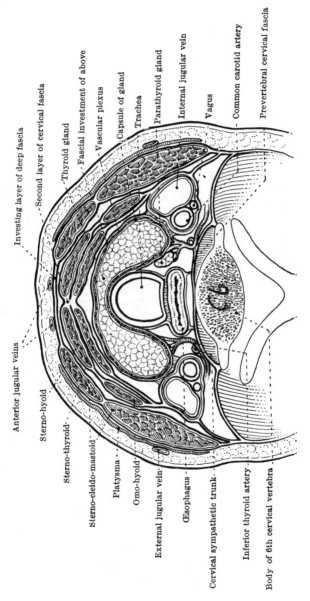

Anterior jugular veins

Investing layer of deep fascia

Second layer of cervical fascia

Thyroid gland

Fascial investment of above

Vascular plexus

Capsule of gland

Trachea

Parathyroid gland

Internal jugular vein

Vagus

Common carotid artery

Prevertebral cervical fascia

Sterno-hyoid

Sterno-thyroid

Sterno-cleido-mastoid

Platysma

Omo-hyoid

External jugular vein

Œsophagus

Cervical sympathetic trunk

Inferior thyroid artery

Body of 6th cervical vertebra

8

PLATE 114.—SUPERFICIAL VEINS OF HEAD

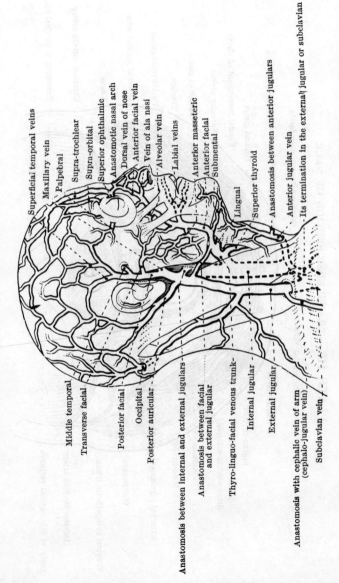

Superficial temporal veins
Maxillary vein
Palpebral
Supra-trochlear
Supra-orbital
Superior ophthalmic
Anastomotic nasal arch
Dorsal vein of nose
Anterior facial vein
Vein of ala nasi
Alveolar vein
Labial veins
Anterior masseteric
Anterior facial
Submental
Lingual
Superior thyroid
Anastomosis between anterior jugulars
Anterior jugular vein
Its termination in the external jugular or subclavian

Middle temporal
Transverse facial
Posterior facial
Occipital
Posterior auricular
Anastomosis between internal and external jugulars
Anastomosis between facial and external jugular
Thyro-linguo-facial venous trunk
Internal jugular
External jugular
Anastomosis with cephalic vein of arm (cephalo-jugular vein)
Subclavian vein

PLATE 115.—SUPERFICIAL NERVES OF NECK AND BACK OF HEAD

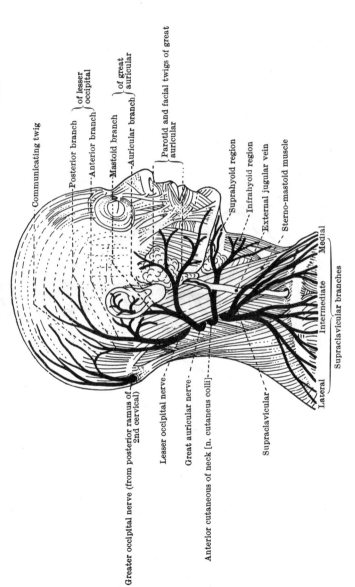

Communicating twig

Posterior branch } of lesser
Anterior branch } occipital

Mastoid branch } of great
Auricular branch } auricular

Parotid and facial twigs of great auricular

Suprahyoid region

Infrahyoid region

External jugular vein

Sterno-mastoid muscle

Medial

Intermediate

Lateral

Supraclavicular branches

Greater occipital nerve (from posterior ramus of 2nd cervical)

Lesser occipital nerve

Great auricular nerve

Anterior cutaneous of neck [n. cutaneus colli]

Supraclavicular

PLATE 116.—ARTERIES OF NECK AND HEAD

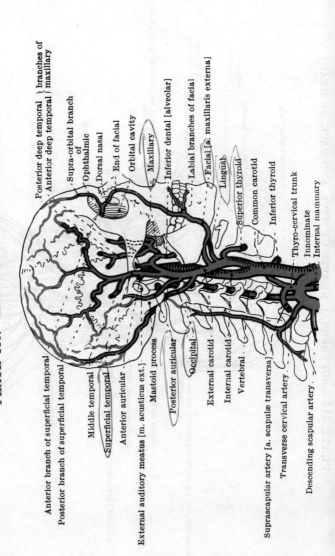

Anterior branch of superficial temporal

Posterior branch of superficial temporal

Middle temporal

Superficial temporal

Anterior auricular

External auditory meatus [m. acusticus ext.]

Mastoid process

Posterior auricular

Occipital

External carotid

Internal carotid

Vertebral

Suprascapular artery [a. scapulae transversa]

Transverse cervical artery

Descending scapular artery

Posterior deep temporal } branches of
Anterior deep temporal } maxillary

Supra-orbital branch of Ophthalmic

Dorsal nasal

End of facial

Orbital cavity

Maxillary

Inferior dental [alveolar]

Labial branches of facial

Facial [a. maxillaris externa]

Lingual

Superior thyroid

Common carotid

Inferior thyroid

Thyro-cervical trunk

Innominate

Internal mammary

PLATE 117.—VASCULAR AND NERVOUS RELATIONS IN NECK

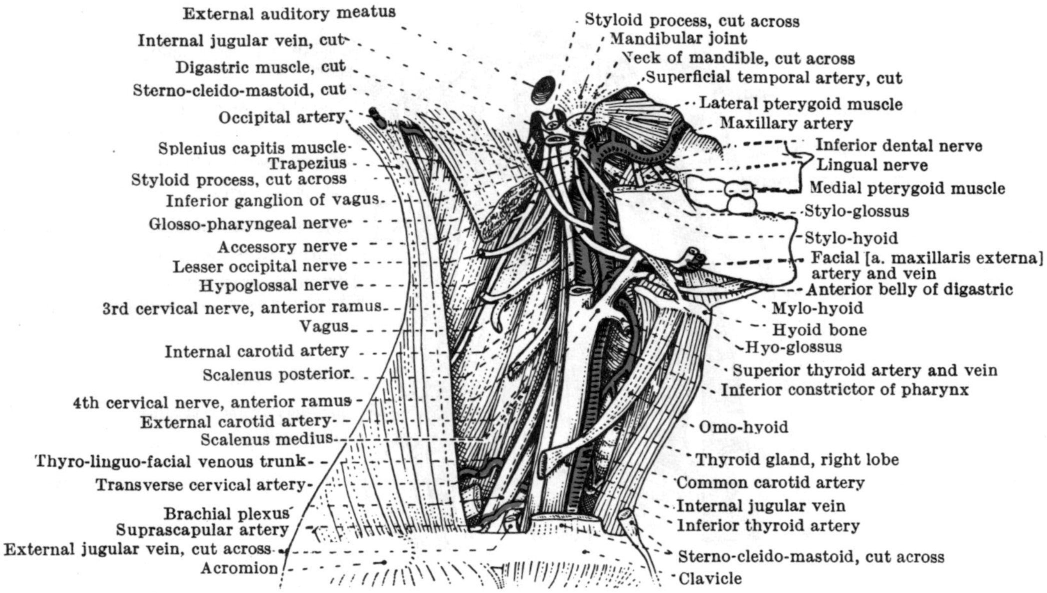

External auditory meatus

Internal jugular vein, cut

Digastric muscle, cut

Sterno-cleido-mastoid, cut

Occipital artery

Splenius capitis muscle
Trapezius
Styloid process, cut across
Inferior ganglion of vagus
Glosso-pharyngeal nerve

Accessory nerve
Lesser occipital nerve
Hypoglossal nerve
Vagus
3rd cervical nerve, anterior ramus

Internal carotid artery
Scalenus posterior

4th cervical nerve, anterior ramus
External carotid artery
Scalenus medius

Thyro-linguo-facial venous trunk
Transverse cervical artery
Brachial plexus
Suprascapular artery
External jugular vein, cut across
Acromion

Styloid process, cut across
Mandibular joint
Neck of mandible, cut across
Superficial temporal artery, cut
Lateral pterygoid muscle
Maxillary artery
Inferior dental nerve
Lingual nerve
Medial pterygoid muscle
Stylo-glossus

Stylo-hyoid
Facial [a. maxillaris externa]
artery and vein
Anterior belly of digastric

Mylo-hyoid
Hyoid bone
Hyo-glossus
Superior thyroid artery and vein
Inferior constrictor of pharynx

Omo-hyoid

Thyroid gland, right lobe
Common carotid artery
Internal jugular vein
Inferior thyroid artery

Sterno-cleido-mastoid, cut across

Clavicle

PLATE 118.—COMMON CAROTID ARTERIES

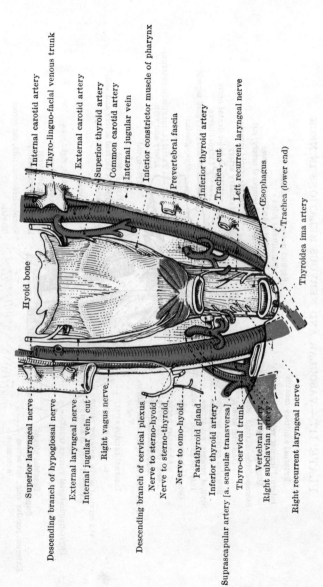

Superior laryngeal nerve

Descending branch of hypoglossal nerve

External laryngeal nerve

Internal jugular vein, cut

Right vagus nerve

Descending branch of cervical plexus

Nerve to sterno-hyoid

Nerve to sterno-thyroid

Nerve to omo-hyoid

Parathyroid gland

Inferior thyroid artery

Suprascapular artery [a. scapulae transversa]

Thyro-cervical trunk

Vertebral artery

Right subclavian artery

Right recurrent laryngeal nerve

Hyoid bone

Internal carotid artery

Thyro-linguo-facial venous trunk

External carotid artery

Superior thyroid artery

Common carotid artery

Internal jugular vein

Inferior constrictor muscle of pharynx

Prevertebral fascia

Inferior thyroid artery

Trachea, cut

Left recurrent laryngeal nerve

Œsophagus

Trachea (lower end)

Thyroidea ima artery

PLATE 119.—SUPERFICIAL ARTERIES OF THE HEAD

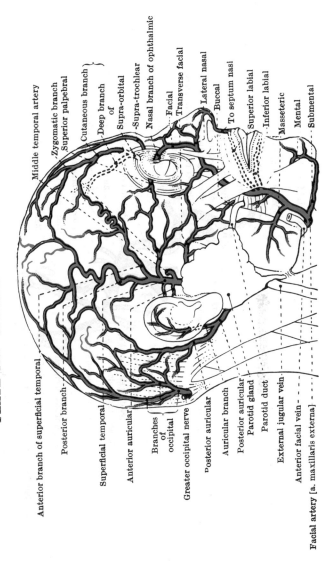

Middle temporal artery

Zygomatic branch
Superior palpebral

Cutaneous branch
Deep branch } of
Supra-orbital

Supra-trochlear

Nasal branch of ophthalmic

Facial
Transverse facial

Lateral nasal

Buccal

To septum nasi

Superior labial

Inferior labial

Masseteric

Mental

Submental

Anterior branch of superficial temporal

Posterior branch

Superficial temporal

Anterior auricular

Branches of occipital

Greater occipital nerve

Posterior auricular

Auricular branch

Posterior auricular

Parotid gland

Parotid duct

External jugular vein

Anterior facial vein

Facial artery [a. maxillaris externa]

PLATE 120.—BRANCHES OF MAXILLARY ARTERY

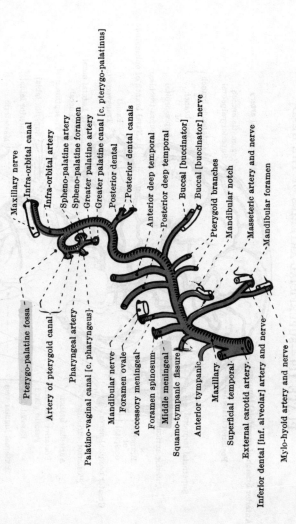

Maxillary nerve

Infra-orbital canal

Infra-orbital artery

Spheno-palatine artery

Spheno-palatine foramen

Greater palatine artery

Greater palatine canal [c. pterygo-palatinus]

Posterior dental

Posterior dental canals

Anterior deep temporal

Posterior deep temporal

Buccal [buccinator]

Buccal [buccinator] nerve

Pterygoid branches

Mandibular notch

Masseteric artery and nerve

Mandibular foramen

Pterygo-palatine fossa

Artery of pterygoid canal

Pharyngeal artery

Palatino-vaginal canal [c. pharyngeus]

Mandibular nerve

Foramen ovale

Accessory meningeal

Foramen spinosum

Middle meningeal

Squamo-tympanic fissure

Anterior tympanic

Maxillary

Superficial temporal

External carotid artery

Inferior dental [Inf. alveolar] artery and nerve

Mylo-hyoid artery and nerve

PLATE 121.—OPHTHALMIC ARTERY—VIEWED FROM ABOVE

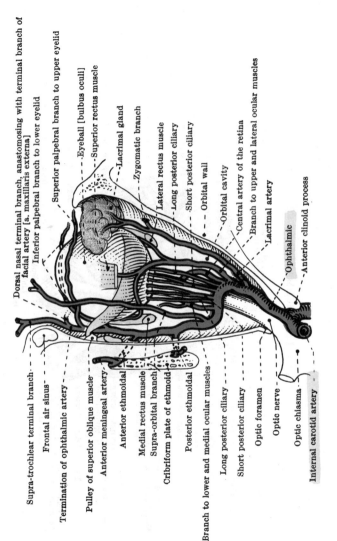

- Dorsal nasal terminal branch, anastomosing with terminal branch of facial artery [a. maxillaris externa]
- Inferior palpebral branch to lower eyelid
- Superior palpebral branch to upper eyelid
- Eyeball [bulbus oculi]
- Superior rectus muscle
- Lacrimal gland
- Zygomatic branch
- Lateral rectus muscle
- Long posterior ciliary
- Short posterior ciliary
- Orbital wall
- Orbital cavity
- Central artery of the retina
- Branch to upper and lateral ocular muscles
- Lacrimal artery
- Ophthalmic
- Anterior clinoid process

- Supra-trochlear terminal branch
- Frontal air sinus
- Termination of ophthalmic artery
- Pulley of superior oblique muscle
- Anterior meningeal artery
- Anterior ethmoidal
- Medial rectus muscle
- Supra-orbital branch
- Cribriform plate of ethmoid
- Posterior ethmoidal
- Branch to lower and medial ocular muscles
- Long posterior ciliary
- Short posterior ciliary
- Optic foramen
- Optic nerve
- Optic chiasma
- Internal carotid artery

PLATE 122.—SUBMANDIBULAR REGION

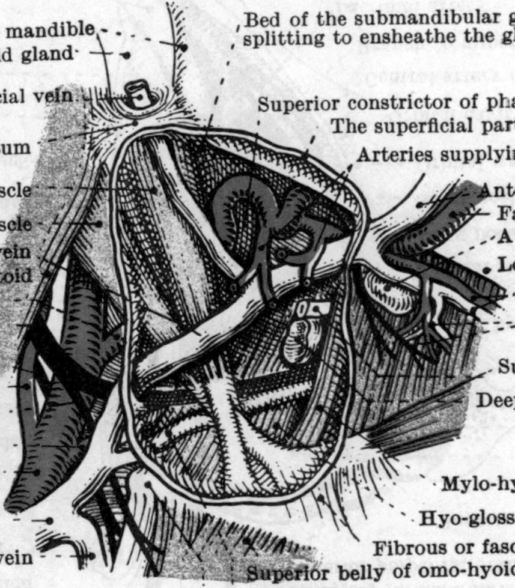

Posterior border of ramus of mandible
Bed of parotid gland

Anterior division of posterior facial vein

Interglandular fascial septum

Stylo-hyoid muscle
Digastric muscle
Common facial vein
Anterior border of sterno-mastoid
Facial artery [a. maxillaris externa]
Hypoglossal nerve

Superior laryngeal nerve
Occipital artery
Special branch of hypoglossal nerve to thyro-hyoid
Lingual artery
External carotid artery

Venous trunk receiving lingual, common facial, and thyroid veins
Superior thyroid vein

Bed of the submandibular gland (the cervical fascia splitting to ensheathe the gland)

Superior constrictor of pharynx
The superficial part of the fascial sheath cut away
Arteries supplying submandibular gland

Anterior facial vein
Facial artery [a. maxillaris externa]
A submandibular lymphatic gland
Lower border of mandible
Submental artery and vein
Vessels and nerves to the mylo-hyoid muscle

Submandibular duct

Deep process of submandibular gland

Mylo-hyoid muscle
Hyo-glossus muscle
Fibrous or fascial band of the digastric muscle
Superior belly of omo-hyoid
Lingual vein
Greater horn of hyoid bone

PLATE 123.—EXTERNAL CAROTID ARTERY

Middle deep temporal artery

Middle deep temporal nerve

Middle and accessory meningeal arteries

Posterior deep temporal nerve

Lateral pterygoid muscle

Middle temporal artery

Auriculo-temporal nerve

Articular artery to mandibular joint

Anterior auricular artery

Facial nerve

Mastoid process

Stylo-mastoid artery

Transverse facial artery

Tympanic artery

Superficial temporal artery

Parotid arteries

Lateral pterygoid arteries

Mylo-hyoid artery and nerve

Posterior auricular artery

Superior constrictor of pharynx

Ascending pharyngeal artery

Occipital artery

Sterno-mastoid muscle

Lingual artery

External carotid artery

Superior thyroid artery

Internal carotid artery

Common carotid artery

Anterior deep temporal artery and nerve

Temporal muscle

Maxillary nerve

Infra-orbital artery

Spheno-palatine, art. of pterygoid canal, pharyngeal, greater palatine arteries

Masseter artery and nerve

Zygomatic arch, cut across

Posterior superior dental artery

Pterygo-maxillary fissure

For communication with facial nerve

Lateral pterygoid artery and nerve

Buccal [buccinator] artery and nerve

Buccinator muscle

Pterygo-mandibular ligament [raphe]

Lingual nerve

Maxillary artery

Inferior dental artery and nerve [a. et n. alveolaris inf.]

Mandible, cut

Facial artery [a. maxillaris externa]

Submental artery

Mylo-hyoid muscle

Hyo-glossus muscle

Hyoid bone

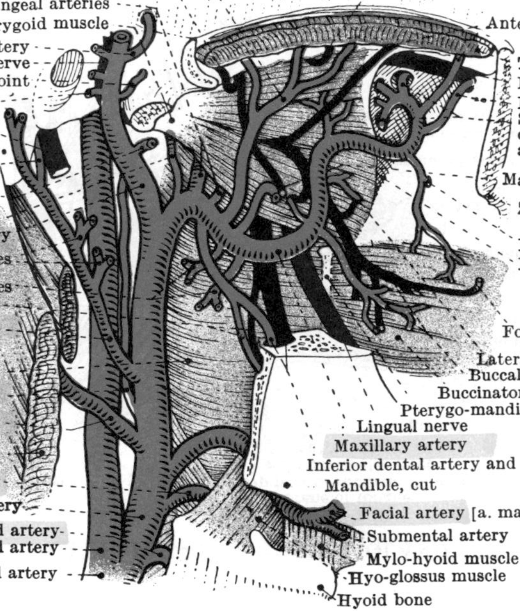

PLATE 124.—SUBLINGUAL GLAND

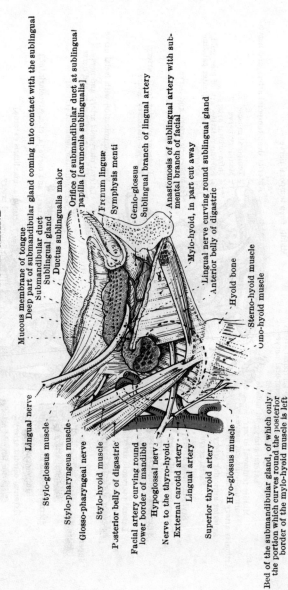

Lingual nerve

Stylo-glossus muscle

Stylo-pharyngeus muscle

Glosso-pharyngeal nerve

Stylo-hyoid muscle

Posterior belly of digastric

Facial artery curving round
lower border of mandible

Hypoglossal nerve

Nerve to the thyro-hyoid

External carotid artery

Lingual artery

Superior thyroid artery

Hyo-glossus muscle

Bed of the submandibular gland, of which only
the portion which curves round the posterior
border of the mylo-hyoid muscle is left

Mucous membrane of tongue
Deep part of submandibular gland coming into contact with the sublingual
Submandibular duct
Sublingual gland
Ductus sublingualis major

Orifice of submandibular duct at sublingual
papilla [caruncula sublingualis]

Frenum linguae
Symphysis menti

Genio-glossus
Sublingual branch of lingual artery

Anastomosis of sublingual artery with submental branch of facial

Mylo-hyoid, in part cut away

Lingual nerve curving round sublingual gland
Anterior belly of digastric

Hyoid bone

Sterno-hyoid muscle
Omo-hyoid muscle

PLATE 125.—VESSELS AND NERVES OF THE TONGUE

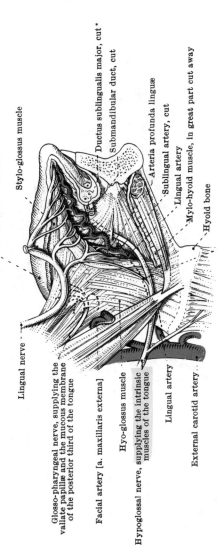

Mucous membrane of tongue, supplied by the lingual nerve in its anterior two-thirds (in front of the V)

Stylo-glossus muscle

Ductus sublingualis major, cut *

Submandibular duct, cut

Arteria profunda linguæ

Sublingual artery, cut

Lingual artery

Mylo-hyoid muscle, in great part cut away

Hyoid bone

Communication between lingual and hypoglossal nerves

Lingual nerve

Glosso-pharyngeal nerve, supplying the vallate papillæ and the mucous membrane of the posterior third of the tongue

Facial artery [a. maxillaris externa]

Hyo-glossus muscle

Hypoglossal nerve, supplying the intrinsic muscles of the tongue

Lingual artery

External carotid artery

* The sublingual gland more frequently opens on to the surface by the ductus sublinguales minores, about 12 in number and of small size. The orifices are serially arranged along the sublingual fold (plica sublingualis).

PLATE 126.—PAROTID REGION

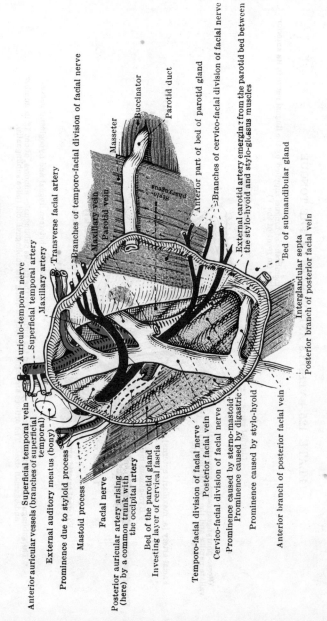

Anterior auricular vessels (branches of superficial temporal)

Superficial temporal vein

Superficial temporal artery

Auriculo-temporal nerve

Maxillary artery

Transverse facial artery

External auditory meatus (bony)

Prominence due to styloid process

Mastoid process

Branches of temporo-facial division of facial nerve

Maxillary vein (Carotid vein)

Posterior facial vein

Masseter

Buccinator

Facial nerve

Mylo-hyoid

Parotid duct

Posterior auricular artery arising (here) by a common trunk with the occipital artery

Anterior part of bed of parotid gland

Bed of the parotid gland

Investing layer of cervical fascia

Branches of cervico-facial division of facial nerve

External carotid artery emerging from the parotid bed between the stylo-hyoid and stylo-glossus muscles

Temporo-facial division of facial nerve

Bed of submandibular gland

Posterior facial vein

Interglandular septa

Cervico-facial division of facial nerve

Posterior branch of posterior facial vein

Prominence caused by sterno-mastoid

Prominence caused by digastric

Prominence caused by stylo-hyoid

Anterior branch of posterior facial vein

PLATE 127.—HORIZONTAL SECTION THROUGH PAROTID REGION

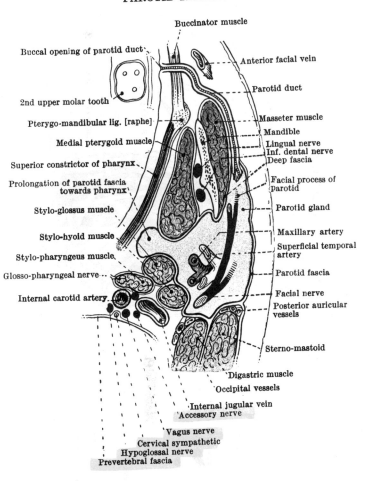

Buccinator muscle

Buccal opening of parotid duct

Anterior facial vein

Parotid duct

2nd upper molar tooth

Masseter muscle

Pterygo-mandibular lig. [raphe]

Mandible

Medial pterygoid muscle

Lingual nerve
Inf. dental nerve
Deep fascia

Superior constrictor of pharynx

Facial process of parotid

Prolongation of parotid fascia towards pharynx

Stylo-glossus muscle

Parotid gland

Stylo-hyoid muscle

Maxillary artery

Stylo-pharyngeus muscle

Superficial temporal artery

Glosso-pharyngeal nerve

Parotid fascia

Internal carotid artery

Facial nerve

Posterior auricular vessels

Sterno-mastoid

Digastric muscle

Occipital vessels

Internal jugular vein
Accessory nerve

Vagus nerve
Cervical sympathetic
Hypoglossal nerve
Prevertebral fascia

PLATE 128.—TONSILLAR REGION

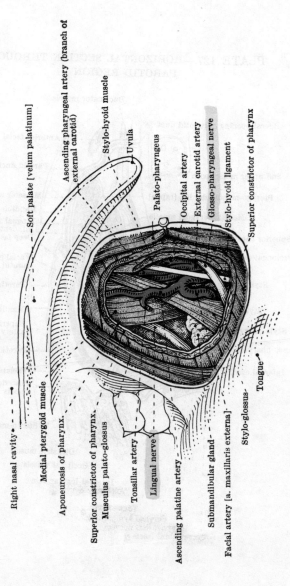

Right nasal cavity

Medial pterygoid muscle

Aponeurosis of pharynx

Superior constrictor of pharynx

Musculus palato-glossus

Tonsillar artery

Lingual nerve

Ascending palatine artery

Submandibular gland

Facial artery [a. maxillaris externa]

Stylo-glossus

Tongue

Soft palate [velum palatinum]

Ascending pharyngeal artery (branch of external carotid)

Stylo-hyoid muscle

Uvula

Palato-pharyngeus

Occipital artery

External carotid artery

Glosso-pharyngeal nerve

Stylo-hyoid ligament

Superior constrictor of pharynx

PLATE 129.—FLOOR OF FOURTH VENTRICLE

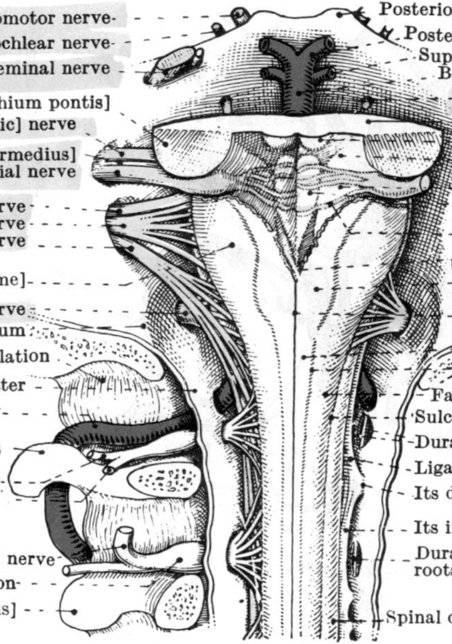

Posterior clinoid process
Posterior cerebral artery
Superior cerebellar artery
Basilar artery
6th or abducent nerve
Pons (cut across)
Eminentia medialis
4th ventricle
Fovea superior
Colliculus facialis
Auditory striæ [s. medullares]
Obex
Gracile tubercle [clava]
Posterior median fissure
Fasciculus gracilis
Paramedian fissure
Fasciculus cuneatus
Sulcus lateralis posterior
Dural openings for spinal nerve roots
Ligamentum denticulatum (of pia mater)
Its denticulations
Its intervening arches
Dural partition separating anterior from posterior nerve roots at their emergence from the cord
Spinal cord [medulla spinalis]

3rd or oculomotor nerve
4th or trochlear nerve
Roots of the 5th or trigeminal nerve

Middle cerebellar peduncle [brachium pontis]
8th or auditory [acoustic] nerve

Sensory root of facial [nervus intermedius]
Motor root of 7th or facial nerve

9th or glosso-pharyngeal nerve
10th or vagus nerve
11th or accessory nerve

Inf. cerebellar peduncle [corpus restiforme]

12th or hypoglossal nerve
Foramen magnum
Occipito-atlantoid articulation
Spinal dura mater
Vertebral artery
Atlas

Anterior ramus of 1st cervical nerve
Posterior ramus of 1st cervical nerve

Posterior ramus of 2nd cervical nerve
Spinal ganglion
Axis [epistropheus]

9

PLATE 130.—ARTERIES OF THE CRANIAL FOSSÆ

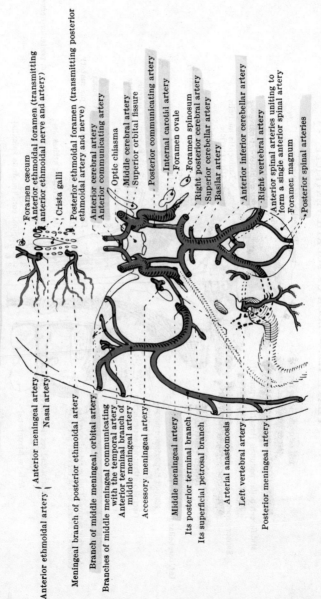

Anterior ethmoidal artery { Anterior meningeal artery / Nasal artery

Meningeal branch of posterior ethmoidal artery

Branch of middle meningeal, orbital artery

Branches of middle meningeal { Anterior terminal branch of middle meningeal artery

Accessory meningeal artery

Middle meningeal artery

Its posterior terminal branch

Its superficial petrosal branch

Arterial anastomosis

Left vertebral artery

Posterior meningeal artery

Foramen cæcum
Anterior ethmoidal foramen (transmitting anterior ethmoidal nerve and artery)
Crista galli
Posterior ethmoidal foramen (transmitting posterior ethmoidal artery and nerve)
Anterior cerebral artery
Anterior communicating artery
Optic chiasma
Middle cerebral artery
Superior orbital fissure
Posterior communicating artery
Internal carotid artery
Foramen ovale
Right posterior cerebral artery
Superior cerebellar artery
Basilar artery
Anterior inferior cerebellar artery
Right vertebral artery
Anterior spinal arteries uniting to form a single anterior spinal artery
Foramen magnum
Posterior spinal arteries

Anterior meningeal communicating with the temporal artery

Foramen spinosum

PLATE 131.—PONS AND MEDULLA OBLONGATA

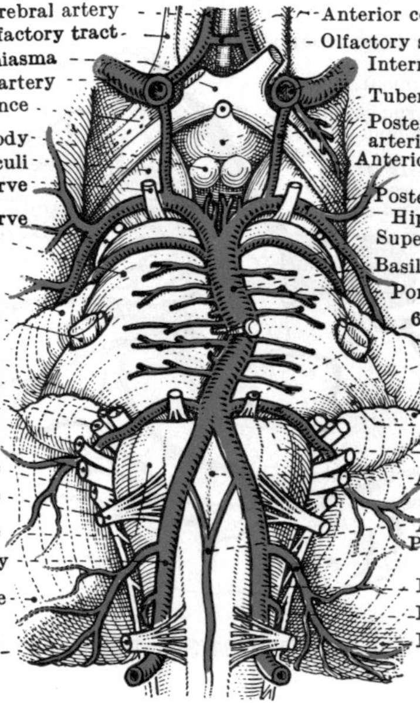

Anterior cerebral artery
Olfactory tract
Optic chiasma
Middle cerebral artery
Anterior perforated substance
Mamillary body
Basis pedunculi
3rd or oculomotor nerve
4th or trochlear nerve
Pons
Cerebellum
5th or trigeminal nerve
7th or facial nerve
Sensory root of 7th [nervus intermedius]
8th or auditory nerve
9th or glosso-pharyngeal nerve
10th or vagus nerve
11th or accessory nerve
12th or hypoglossal nerve
Olive
Right vertebral artery
Right cerebellar hemisphere
Anterior or motor root of 1st spinal nerve

Anterior communicating artery
Olfactory sulcus
Internal carotid artery
Tuber cinereum
Posterior communicating artery completing circulus arteriosus
Anterior choroidal artery
Posterior cerebral artery
Hippocampus
Superior cerebellar artery
Basilar artery
Pontine arteries
6th or abducent nerve
Anterior inferior cerebellar artery
Flocculus
Middle cerebellar peduncle [brachium pontis]
Pontine sulcus
Anterior median fissure of medulla
Anterior spinal artery
Posterior inferior cerebellar artery
Left vertebral artery
Posterior spinal artery
Left cerebellar hemisphere

PLATE 132.—CEREBRAL AND CEREBELLAR CIRCULATION—MEDIAL VIEW

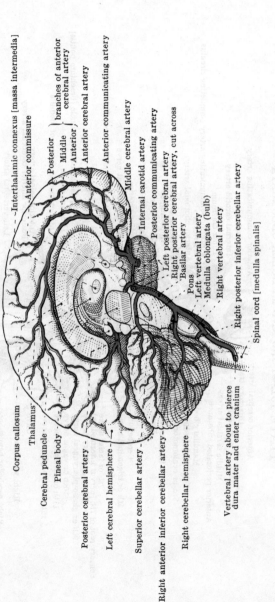

Corpus callosum
Thalamus
Cerebral peduncle
Pineal body

Posterior cerebral artery
Left cerebral hemisphere

Superior cerebellar artery

Right anterior inferior cerebellar artery

Right cerebellar hemisphere

Vertebral artery about to pierce
dura mater and enter cranium

Interthalamic connexus [massa intermedia]
Anterior commissure

Posterior
Middle   } branches of anterior
Anterior   cerebral artery
Anterior cerebral artery

Anterior communicating artery

Middle cerebral artery

Internal carotid artery

Posterior communicating artery
Left posterior cerebral artery
Right posterior cerebral artery, cut across
Basilar artery
Pons
Left vertebral artery
Medulla oblongata (bulb)
Right vertebral artery

Right posterior inferior cerebellar artery

Spinal cord [medulla spinalis]

PLATE 133.—CEREBRAL AND CEREBELLAR CIRCULATION—SEEN FROM BELOW

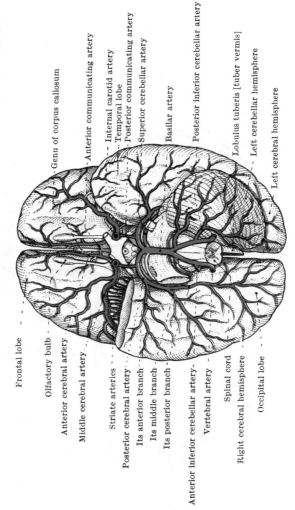

Frontal lobe

Olfactory bulb

Anterior cerebral artery

Middle cerebral artery

Striate arteries

Posterior cerebral artery

Its anterior branch

Its middle branch

Its posterior branch

Anterior inferior cerebellar artery

Vertebral artery

Spinal cord

Right cerebral hemisphere

Occipital lobe

Genu of corpus callosum

Anterior communicating artery

Internal carotid artery

Temporal lobe

Posterior communicating artery

Superior cerebellar artery

Basilar artery

Posterior inferior cerebellar artery

Lobulus tuberis [tuber vermis]

Left cerebellar hemisphere

Left cerebral hemisphere

PLATE 134.—MEDIAN SECTION OF HEAD

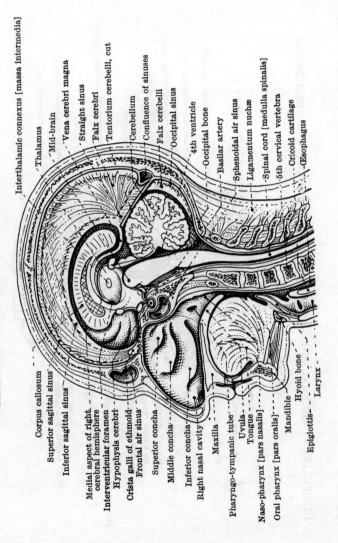

Interthalamic connexus [massa intermedia]
Thalamus
Mid-brain
Vena cerebri magna
Straight sinus
Falx cerebri
Tentorium cerebelli, cut
Cerebellum
Confluence of sinuses
Falx cerebelli
Occipital sinus
4th ventricle
Occipital bone
Basilar artery
Sphenoidal air sinus
Ligamentum nuchae
Spinal cord [medulla spinalis]
5th cervical vertebra
Cricoid cartilage
Œsophagus

Corpus callosum
Superior sagittal sinus
Inferior sagittal sinus
Medial aspect of right cerebral hemisphere
Interventricular foramen
Hypophysis cerebri
Crista galli of ethmoid
Frontal air sinus
Superior concha
Middle concha
Inferior concha
Right nasal cavity
Maxilla
Pharyngo-tympanic tube
Uvula
Tongue
Naso-pharynx [pars nasalis]
Oral pharynx [pars oralis]
Mandible
Hyoid bone
Epiglottis
Larynx

PLATE 135.—LARYNX

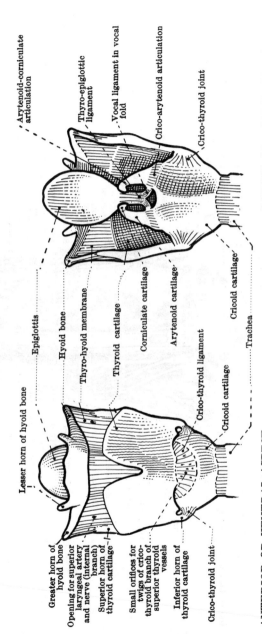

Labels (anterior figure, left):
- Lesser horn of hyoid bone
- Greater horn of hyoid bone
- Opening for superior laryngeal artery and nerve (internal branch)
- Superior horn of thyroid cartilage
- Small orifices for twigs of crico-thyroid branch of superior thyroid vessels
- Inferior horn of thyroid cartilage
- Crico-thyroid joint

Labels (centre):
- Epiglottis
- Hyoid bone
- Thyro-hyoid membrane
- Thyroid cartilage
- Corniculate cartilage
- Arytenoid cartilage
- Crico-thyroid ligament
- Cricoid cartilage
- Trachea

Labels (dorsal figure, right):
- Arytenoid-corniculate articulation
- Thyro-epiglottic ligament
- Vocal ligament in vocal fold
- Crico-arytenoid articulation
- Crico-thyroid joint
- Cricoid cartilage

ANTERIOR OR VENTRAL ASPECT

DORSAL OR POSTERIOR ASPECT

PLATE 136.—PHARYNX AND ITS RELATIONS

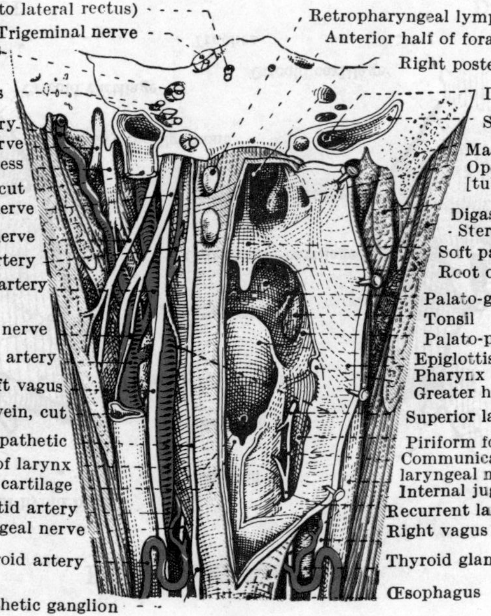

Abducent nerve (to lateral rectus)
Trigeminal nerve
Facial and auditory nerves
Retropharyngeal lymph glands
Anterior half of foramen magnum
Right posterior aperture of nose [choana]
Internal jugular vein
Sigmoid sinus
Mastoid process
Opening of the pharyngo-tympanic tube [tuba auditiva]
Digastric muscle, cut
Sterno-cleido-mastoid
Soft palate
Root of tongue
Palato-glossal arch
Tonsil
Palato-pharyngeal arch
Epiglottis
Pharynx
Greater horn of hyoid bone
Superior laryngeal nerves
Piriform fossa
Communication between superior and recurrent laryngeal nerves
Internal jugular vein
Recurrent laryngeal nerve
Right vagus
Thyroid gland
Œsophagus

Glosso-pharyngeal, vagus, and accessory nerves
Occipital artery
Facial nerve
Styloid process
Internal jugular vein, cut
Hypoglossal nerve
Accessory nerve
Ascending pharyngeal artery
Internal carotid artery
Descending branch of hypoglossal nerve
External carotid artery
Left vagus
Internal jugular vein, cut
Cervical sympathetic
Cavity of larynx
Left arytenoid cartilage
Common carotid artery
Left recurrent laryngeal nerve
Inferior thyroid artery
Middle cervical sympathetic ganglion

PLATE 137.—MEDIAN SECTION OF NECK

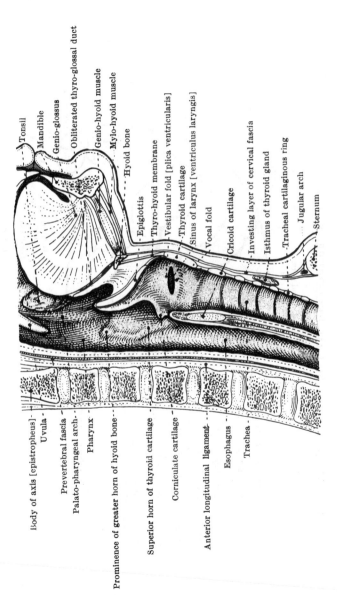

Tonsil
Mandible
Genio-glossus
Obliterated thyro-glossal duct
Genio-hyoid muscle
Mylo-hyoid muscle
Hyoid bone
Epiglottis
Thyro-hyoid membrane
Vestibular fold [plica ventricularis]
Thyroid cartilage
Sinus of larynx [ventriculus laryngis]
Vocal fold
Cricoid cartilage
Investing layer of cervical fascia
Isthmus of thyroid gland
Tracheal cartilaginous ring
Jugular arch
Sternum

Body of axis [epistropheus]
Uvula
Prevertebral fascia
Palato-pharyngeal arch
Pharynx
Prominence of greater horn of hyoid bone
Superior horn of thyroid cartilage
Corniculate cartilage
Anterior longitudinal ligament
Esophagus
Trachea

PLATE 138.—LEFT CEREBRAL HEMISPHERE—SUPERO-LATERAL SURFACE

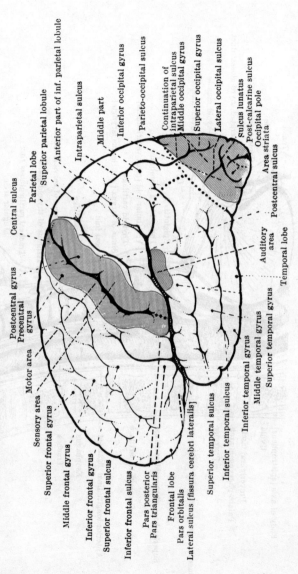

Central sulcus

Postcentral gyrus
Precentral
gyrus

Parietal lobe
Superior parietal lobule
Anterior part of inf. parietal lobule

Intraparietal sulcus

Middle part

Inferior occipital gyrus

Parieto-occipital sulcus

Continuation of
intraparietal sulcus
Middle occipital gyrus

Superior occipital gyrus

Lateral occipital sulcus

sulcus lunatus
Post-calcarine sulcus
Occipital pole

Area striata

Postcentral sulcus

Auditory
area

Temporal lobe

Sensory area

Motor area

Superior frontal gyrus

Middle frontal gyrus

Inferior frontal gyrus

Superior frontal sulcus

Inferior frontal sulcus

Pars posterior
Pars triangularis

Frontal lobe

Pars orbitalis

Lateral sulcus [fissura cerebri lateralis]

Superior temporal sulcus

Inferior temporal sulcus

Inferior temporal gyrus
Middle temporal gyrus
Superior temporal gyrus

The red shaded region in occipital lobe represents the visual area.

PLATE 139.—LEFT CEREBRAL HEMISPHERE—MEDIAL ASPECT

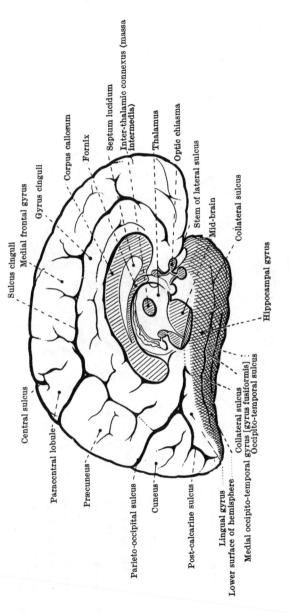

Central sulcus

Paracentral lobule

Præcuneus

Parieto-occipital sulcus

Cuneus

Post-calcarine sulcus

Lingual gyrus
Lower surface of hemisphere
Medial occipito-temporal gyrus [gyrus fusiformis] :
Occipito-temporal sulcus

Collateral sulcus

Sulcus cinguli
Medial frontal gyrus
Gyrus cinguli
Corpus callosum
Fornix
Septum lucidum
Inter-thalamic connexus (massa intermedia)
Thalamus
Optic chiasma
Stem of lateral sulcus
Mid-brain
Collateral sulcus
Hippocampal gyrus

PLATE 140.—CORONAL SECTION OF BRAIN (SLIGHTLY OBLIQUE) THROUGH CEREBRUM, MID-BRAIN AND PONS

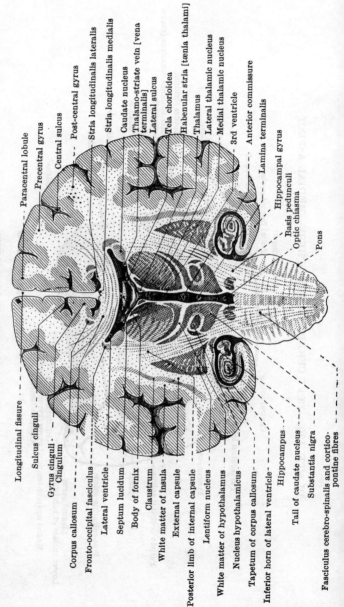

Longitudinal fissure
Sulcus cinguli
Gyrus cinguli
Cingulum
Corpus callosum
Fronto-occipital fasciculus
Lateral ventricle
Septum lucidum
Body of fornix
Claustrum
White matter of insula
External capsule
Posterior limb of internal capsule
Lentiform nucleus
White matter of hypothalamus
Nucleus hypothalamicus
Tapetum of corpus callosum
Inferior horn of lateral ventricle
Tail of caudate nucleus
Substantia nigra
Fasciculus cerebro-spinalis and cortico-pontine fibres

Paracentral lobule
Precentral gyrus
Central sulcus
Post-central gyrus
Stria longitudinalis lateralis
Stria longitudinalis medialis
Caudate nucleus
Thalamo-striate vein [vena terminalis]
Tela chorioidea
Habenular stria [tænia thalami]
Thalamus
Lateral thalamic nucleus
Medial thalamic nucleus
3rd ventricle
Anterior commissure
Lamina terminalis
Hippocampal gyrus
Basis pedunculi
Optic chiasma
Pons
Hippocampus

PLATE 141.—CORONAL SECTION OF BRAIN (OBLIQUE) THROUGH CEREBRUM, BRAIN-STEM AND CEREBELLUM

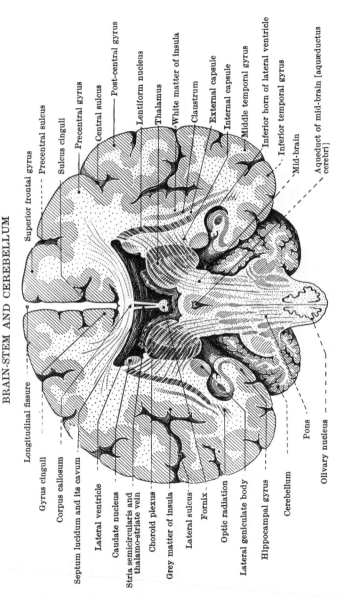

Longitudinal fissure

Superior frontal gyrus

Precentral sulcus

Sulcus cinguli

Precentral gyrus

Central sulcus

Post-central gyrus

Lentiform nucleus

Thalamus

White matter of insula

Claustrum

External capsule

Internal capsule

Middle temporal gyrus

Inferior temporal gyrus

Inferior horn of lateral ventricle

Mid-brain

Aqueduct of mid-brain [aquaeductus cerebri]

Gyrus cinguli

Corpus callosum

Septum lucidum and its cavum

Lateral ventricle

Caudate nucleus

Stria semicircularis and thalamo-striate vein

Choroid plexus

Grey matter of insula

Lateral sulcus

Fornix

Optic radiation

Lateral geniculate body

Hippocampal gyrus

Cerebellum

Pons

Olivary nucleus

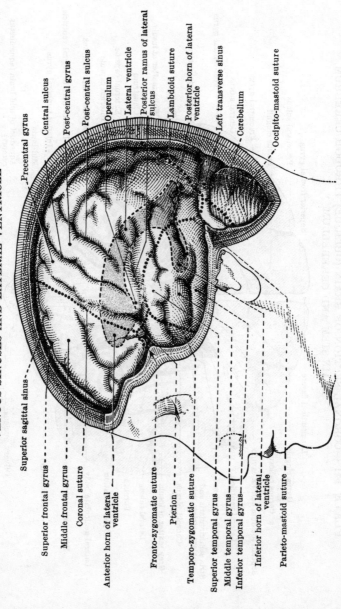

PLATE 142.—RELATIONS OF LEFT CEREBRAL HEMISPHERE TO SUTURES, VENOUS SINUSES AND LATERAL VENTRICLE

Precentral gyrus
Central sulcus
Post-central gyrus
Post-central sulcus
Operculum
Lateral ventricle
Posterior ramus of lateral sulcus
Lambdoid suture
Posterior horn of lateral ventricle
Left transverse sinus
Cerebellum
Occipito-mastoid suture

Superior sagittal sinus
Superior frontal gyrus
Middle frontal gyrus
Coronal suture
Anterior horn of lateral ventricle
Fronto-zygomatic suture
Pterion
Temporo-zygomatic suture
Superior temporal gyrus
Middle temporal gyrus
Inferior temporal gyrus
Inferior horn of lateral ventricle
Parieto-mastoid suture

PLATE 143.—SECTION OF THE RIGHT CEREBRAL HEMISPHERE SHOWING POSITION OF LATERAL VENTRICLE

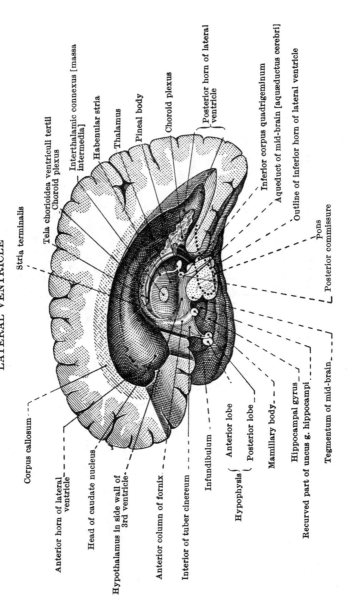

Stria terminalis

Tela chorioidea ventriculi tertii
Choroid plexus

Interthalamic connexus [massa intermedia]

Habenular stria

Thalamus

Pineal body

Choroid plexus

Posterior horn of lateral ventricle

Inferior corpus quadrigeminum

Aqueduct of mid-brain [aqueductus cerebri]

Outline of inferior horn of lateral ventricle

Pons

Posterior commissure

Tegmentum of mid-brain

Hippocampal gyrus

Recurved part of uncus g. hippocampi

Mamillary body

Posterior lobe

Hypophysis {
Anterior lobe

Infundibulum

Interior of tuber cinereum

Anterior column of fornix.

Hypothalamus in side wall of 3rd ventricle

Head of caudate nucleus

Anterior horn of lateral ventricle

Corpus callosum

PLATE 144.—CEREBRUM AND CEREBELLUM—INFERIOR ASPECT

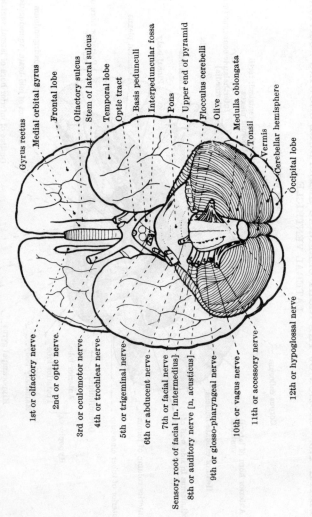

Gyrus rectus

Medial orbital gyrus

Frontal lobe

Olfactory sulcus

Stem of lateral sulcus

Temporal lobe

Optic tract

Basis pedunculi

Interpeduncular fossa

Pons

Upper end of pyramid

Flocculus cerebelli

Olive

Medulla oblongata

Tonsil

Vermis

Cerebellar hemisphere

Occipital lobe

1st or olfactory nerve

2nd or optic nerve

3rd or oculomotor nerve

4th or trochlear nerve

5th or trigeminal nerve

6th or abducent nerve

7th or facial nerve

Sensory root of facial [n. intermedius]

8th or auditory nerve [n. acusticus]

9th or glosso-pharyngeal nerve

10th or vagus nerve

11th or accessory nerve

12th or hypoglossal nerve

PLATE 145.—APERTURES IN BASE OF SKULL

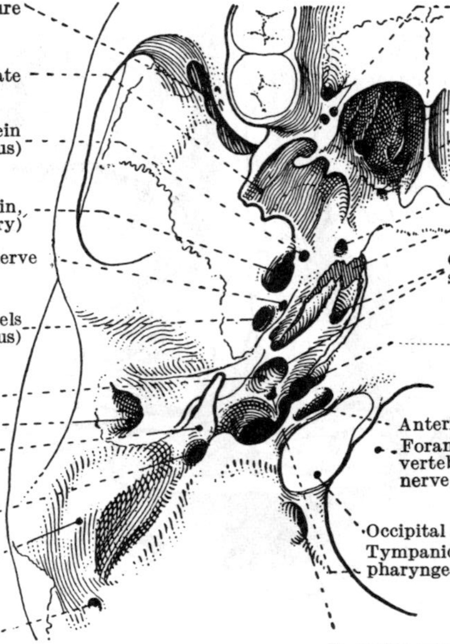

- Inferior orbital fissure
- Lateral pterygoid plate
- Sphenoidal emissary foramen (Vesalius) (for vein between cavernous sinus and pterygoid plexus)
- Foramen ovale (mandibular nerve, emissary vein, and accessory meningeal artery)
- Foramen for lesser superficial petrosal nerve
- Foramen spinosum (for middle meningeal vessels and nervus spinosus)
- Canaliculus carotico-tympanicus (for tympanic branches of internal carotid artery and of carotid sympathetic plexus)
- External auditory meatus
- Styloid process
- Stylo-mastoid foramen for facial nerve and stylo-mastoid artery
- Mastoid process
- Mastoid foramen (for mastoid emissary vein)

- Greater and lesser palatine foramina (for greater and lesser palatine vessels and nerves)
- Posterior aperture of nose [choana]
- Palatino-vaginal canal [c. pharyngeus] for branch of spheno-palatine ganglion and vessels
- Pterygoid canal for nerve and artery of pterygoid canal
- Foramen lacerum
- Carotid canal for internal carotid artery, sympathetic carotid plexus and veins
- Jugular foramen for glosso-pharyngeal, vagus, and accessory nerves, internal jugular vein, inferior petrosal sinus, and meningeal arteries
- Anterior condylar canal [c. hypoglossi]
- Foramen magnum (for spinal cord and membranes, vertebral and spinal arteries, spinal part of accessory nerve)
- Occipital condyle
- Tympanic canaliculus for tympanic branch of glosso-pharyngeal nerve
- Posterior condylar canal for posterior condylar vein

10

PLATE 146.—FLOOR OF FOURTH VENTRICLE

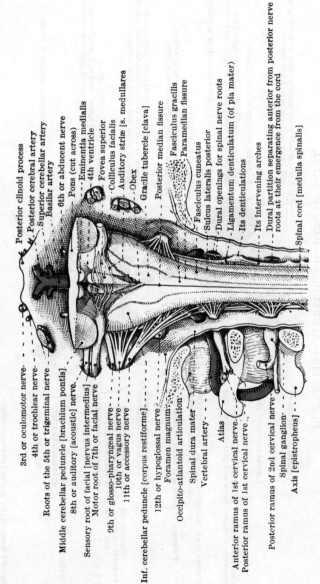

3rd or oculomotor nerve
4th or trochlear nerve
Roots of the 5th or trigeminal nerve
Middle cerebellar peduncle [brachium pontis]
8th or auditory [acoustic] nerve
Sensory root of facial [nervus intermedius]
Motor root of 7th or facial nerve
9th or glosso-pharyngeal nerve
10th or vagus nerve
11th or accessory nerve
Inf. cerebellar peduncle [corpus restiforme]
12th or hypoglossal nerve
Foramen magnum:
Occipito-atlantoid articulation
Spinal dura mater
Vertebral artery
Atlas
Anterior ramus of 1st cervical nerve
Posterior ramus of 1st cervical nerve
Posterior ramus of 2nd cervical nerve
Spinal ganglion
Axis [epistropheus]

Posterior clinoid process
Posterior cerebral artery
Superior cerebellar artery
Basilar artery
6th or abducent nerve
Pons (cut across)
Eminentia medialis
4th ventricle
Fovea superior
Colliculus facialis
Auditory striæ [s. medullares]
Obex
Gracile tubercle [clava]
Posterior median fissure
Fasciculus gracilis
Paramedian fissure
Fasciculus cuneatus
Sulcus lateralis posterior
Dural openings for spinal nerve roots
Ligamentum denticulatum (of pia mater)
Its denticulations
Its intervening arches
Dural partition separating anterior from posterior nerve roots at their emergence from the cord
Spinal cord [medulla spinalis]

PLATE 147.—VENOUS SINUSES OF THE BASE OF THE CRANIUM

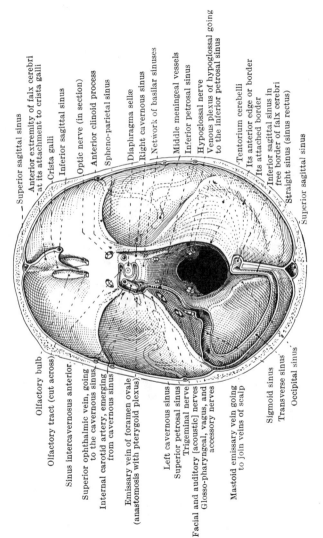

Superior sagittal sinus

Anterior extremity of falx cerebri at its attachment to crista galli

Crista galli

Inferior sagittal sinus

Optic nerve (in section)

Anterior clinoid process

Spheno-parietal sinus

Diaphragma sellæ

Right cavernous sinus

Network of basilar sinuses

Middle meningeal vessels

Inferior petrosal sinus

Hypoglossal nerve

Venous plexus of hypoglossal going to the inferior petrosal sinus

Tentorium cerebelli

Its anterior edge or border

Its attached border

Inferior sagittal sinus in free border of falx cerebri

Straight sinus (sinus rectus)

Superior sagittal sinus

Olfactory bulb

Olfactory tract (cut across)

Sinus intercavernosus anterior

Superior ophthalmic vein, going to the cavernous sinus

Internal carotid artery, emerging from cavernous sinus

Emissary vein of foramen ovale (anastomosis with pterygoid plexus)

Left cavernous sinus

Superior petrosal sinus

Trigeminal nerve

Facial and auditory [acoustic] nerves

Glosso-pharyngeal, vagus, and accessory nerves

Mastoid emissary vein going to join veins of scalp

Sigmoid sinus

Transverse sinus

Occipital sinus

PLATE 148.—NERVES TO THE MUSCLES OF THE EYEBALL: OCULOMOTOR (III), TROCHLEAR (IV), & ABDUCENT (VI)

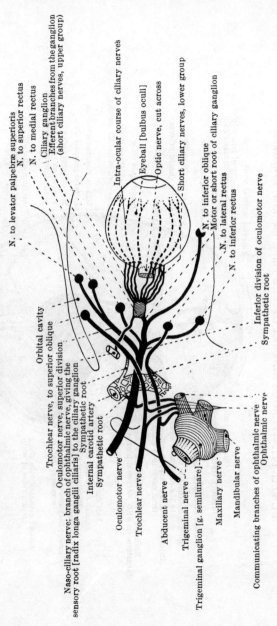

N. to levator palpebræ superioris
N. to superior rectus
N. to medial rectus
Ciliary ganglion
Efferent branches from the ganglion (short ciliary nerves, upper group)
Intra-ocular course of ciliary nerves
Eyeball [bulbus oculi]
Optic nerve, cut across
Short ciliary nerves, lower group
N. to inferior oblique
Motor or short root of ciliary ganglion
N. to lateral rectus
N. to inferior rectus
Inferior division of oculomotor nerve
Sympathetic root

Orbital cavity
Trochlear nerve, to superior oblique
Oculomotor nerve, superior division
Naso-ciliary nerve: branch of ophthalmic nerve, giving the sensory root [radix longa ganglii ciliaris] to the ciliary ganglion
Sympathetic root
Internal carotid artery
Sympathetic root

Oculomotor nerve
Trochlear nerve
Abducent nerve
Trigeminal nerve
Trigeminal ganglion [g. semilunare]
Maxillary nerve
Mandibular nerve
Communicating branches of ophthalmic nerve
Ophthalmic nerve

PLATE 149.—TRIGEMINAL NERVE—OPHTHALMIC DIVISION

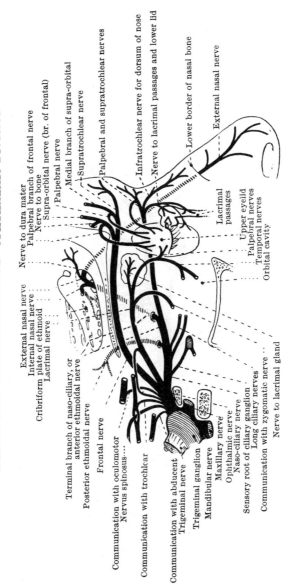

External nasal nerve
Internal nasal nerve
Cribriform plate of ethmoid
Lacrimal nerve

Terminal branch of naso-ciliary, or
anterior ethmoidal nerve
Posterior ethmoidal nerve

Frontal nerve

Communication with oculomotor
Nervus spinosus

Communication with trochlear

Communication with abducent
Trigeminal nerve
Trigeminal ganglion
Mandibular nerve
Maxillary nerve
Ophthalmic nerve
Naso-ciliary nerve
Sensory root of ciliary ganglion
Long ciliary nerves
Communication with zygomatic nerve
Nerve to lacrimal gland

Nerve to dura mater
Palpebral branch of frontal nerve
Nerve to bone
Supra-orbital nerve (br. of frontal)
Palpebral nerve
Medial branch of supra-orbital
Supratrochlear nerve
Palpebral and supratrochlear nerves
Infratrochlear nerve for dorsum of nose
Nerve to lacrimal passages and lower lid
Lower border of nasal bone
External nasal nerve

Lacrimal
passages
Upper eyelid
Palpebral nerves
Temporal nerves
Orbital cavity

PLATE 150.—TRIGEMINAL NERVE—MAXILLARY DIVISION

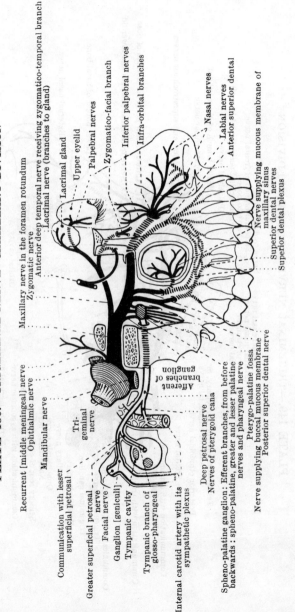

Recurrent [middle meningeal] nerve
Ophthalmic nerve
Mandibular nerve
Maxillary nerve in the foramen rotundum
Zygomatic nerve
Anterior deep temporal nerve receiving zygomatico-temporal branch
Lacrimal nerve (branches to gland)
Lacrimal gland
Upper eyelid
Palpebral nerves
Zygomatico-facial branch
Inferior palpebral nerves
Infra-orbital branches
Nasal nerves
Labial nerves
Anterior superior dental

Communication with lesser superficial petrosal
Greater superficial petrosal nerve
Facial nerve
Ganglion [geniculi]
Tympanic cavity
Tri-geminal nerve

Tympanic branch of glosso-pharyngeal
Internal carotid artery with its sympathetic plexus

Afferent branches of ganglion

Deep petrosal nerve
Nerves of pterygoid cana
Spheno-palatine ganglion: Efferent branches, from before backwards: spheno-palatine, greater and lesser palatine nerves and pharyngeal nerve
Pterygo-palatine fossa
Nerve supplying buccal mucous membrane
Posterior superior dental nerve

Nerve supplying mucous membrane of maxillary sinus
Superior dental nerves
Superior dental plexus

PLATE 151.—TRIGEMINAL NERVE—MAXILLARY DIVISION (*Continued*)

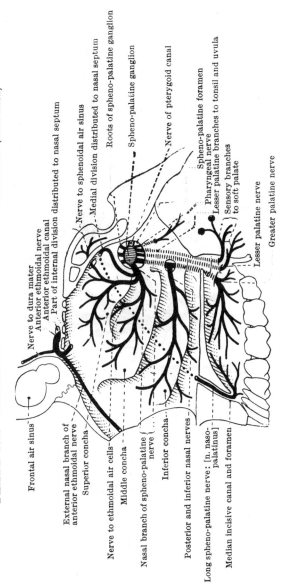

Frontal air sinus

Nerve to dura mater
Anterior ethmoidal nerve
Anterior ethmoidal canal
Part of internal division distributed to nasal septum

Nerve to sphenoidal air sinus
Medial division distributed to nasal septum
Roots of spheno-palatine ganglion
Spheno-palatine ganglion

Nerve of pterygoid canal

External nasal branch of anterior ethmoidal nerve
Superior concha

Nerve to ethmoidal air cells
Middle concha

Nasal branch of spheno-palatine nerve {
Inferior concha

Posterior and inferior nasal nerves

Long spheno-palatine nerve: [n. naso-palatinus]

Median incisive canal and foramen

Spheno-palatine foramen
Pharyngeal nerve
Lesser palatine branches to tonsil and uvula
Sensory branches to soft palate }

Lesser palatine nerve

Greater palatine nerve

PLATE 152.—TRIGEMINAL NERVE—MANDIBULAR DIVISION

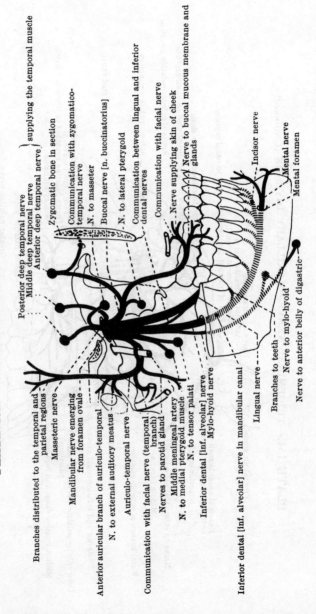

Posterior deep temporal nerve
Middle deep temporal nerve } supplying the temporal muscle
Anterior deep temporal nerve
Zygomatic bone in section
Communication with zygomatico-temporal nerve
N. to masseter
Buccal nerve [n. buccinatorius]
N. to lateral pterygoid
Communication between lingual and inferior dental nerves
Communication with facial nerve
Nerve supplying skin of cheek
Nerve to buccal mucous membrane and glands

Incisor nerve
Mental nerve
Mental foramen

Branches distributed to the temporal and parietal regions
Masseteric nerve

Mandibular nerve emerging from foramen ovale
Anterior auricular branch of auriculo-temporal
Auriculo-temporal nerve

Communication with facial nerve (temporal branch)
Nerves to parotid gland
Middle meningeal artery
N. to medial pterygoid muscle
N. to tensor palati
Inferior dental [inf. alveolar] nerve
Mylo-hyoid nerve

Inferior dental [inf. alveolar] nerve in mandibular canal
Lingual nerve
Branches to teeth
Nerve to mylo-hyoid
Nerve to anterior belly of digastric

PLATE 153.—INFERIOR DENTAL NERVE

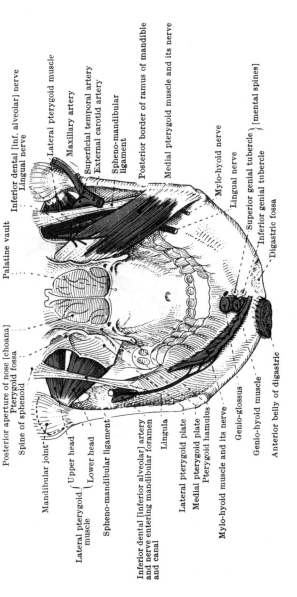

Palatine vault

Inferior dental [inf. alveolar] nerve
Lingual nerve

Lateral pterygoid muscle

Maxillary artery

Superficial temporal artery
External carotid artery

Spheno-mandibular ligament

Posterior border of ramus of mandible

Medial pterygoid muscle and its nerve

Mylo-hyoid nerve

Lingual nerve

Superior genial tubercle ⎫ [mental spines]
Inferior genial tubercle ⎭

Digastric fossa

Posterior aperture of nose [choana]
Pterygoid fossa
Spine of sphenoid

Mandibular joint

Lateral pterygoid ⎰ Upper head
muscle ⎱ Lower head

Spheno-mandibular ligament

Inferior dental [inferior alveolar] artery
and nerve entering mandibular foramen
and canal

Lingula

Lateral pterygoid plate
Medial pterygoid plate
Pterygoid hamulus

Mylo-hyoid muscle and its nerve

Genio-glossus

Genio-hyoid muscle

Anterior belly of digastric

PLATE 154.—MANDIBULAR NERVE (Continued)

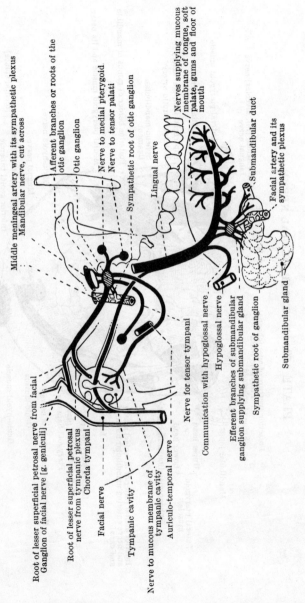

Root of lesser superficial petrosal nerve from facial
Ganglion of facial nerve [g. geniculi]

Root of lesser superficial petrosal nerve from tympanic plexus
Chorda tympani

Facial nerve

Tympanic cavity

Nerve to mucous membrane of tympanic cavity
Auriculo-temporal nerve

Nerve for tensor tympani

Communication with hypoglossal nerve
Hypoglossal nerve

Efferent branches of submandibular ganglion supplying submandibular gland

Sympathetic root of ganglion

Submandibular gland

Middle meningeal artery with its sympathetic plexus
Mandibular nerve, cut across

Afferent branches or roots of the otic ganglion
Otic ganglion

Nerve to medial pterygoid
Nerve to tensor palati

Sympathetic root of otic ganglion

Lingual nerve

Nerves supplying mucous membrane of tongue, soft palate, gums and floor of mouth

Submandibular duct

Facial artery and its sympathetic plexus

PLATE 155.—FACIAL NERVE

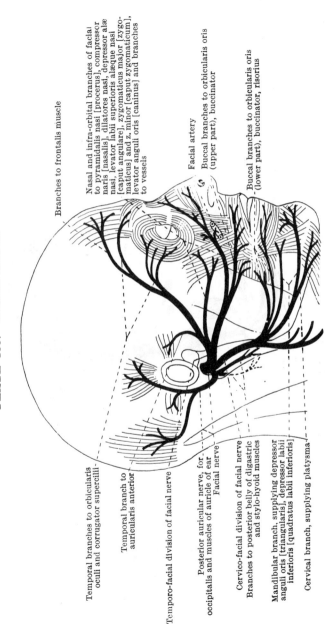

Branches to frontalis muscle

Nasal and infra-orbital branches of facial to pyramidalis nasi [procerus], compressor naris [nasalis], dilatores nasi, depressor alae nasi, levator labii superioris alæque nasi [caput angulare], zygomaticus major [zygomaticus] and z. minor [caput zygomaticum], levator anguli oris [caninus] and branches to vessels

Facial artery

Buccal branches to orbicularis oris (upper part), buccinator

Buccal branches to orbicularis oris (lower part), buccinator, risorius

Temporal branches to orbicularis oculi and corrugator supercilii

Temporal branch to auricularis anterior

Temporo-facial division of facial nerve

Posterior auricular nerve, for occipitalis and muscles of auricle of ear
Facial nerve

Cervico-facial division of facial nerve
Branches to posterior belly of digastric and stylo-hyoid muscles

Mandibular branch, supplying depressor anguli oris [triangularis], depressor labii inferioris [quadratus labii inferioris]

Cervical branch, supplying platysma

PLATE 156.—GLOSSO-PHARYNGEAL NERVE

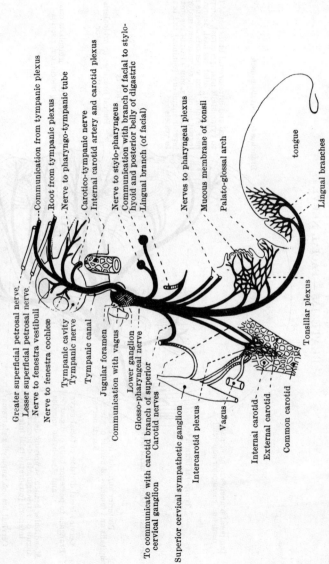

Greater superficial petrosal nerve.
Lesser superficial petrosal nerve.
Nerve to fenestra vestibuli
Nerve to fenestra cochleae

Tympanic cavity
Tympanic nerve
Tympanic canal

Jugular foramen
Communication with vagus
Lower ganglion
Glosso-pharyngeal nerve

To communicate with carotid branch of superior
cervical ganglion
Carotid nerves

Superior cervical sympathetic ganglion

Intercarotid plexus

Vagus

Internal carotid
External carotid

Common carotid

Communication from tympanic plexus
Root from tympanic plexus
Nerve to pharyngo-tympanic tube

Carotico-tympanic nerve
Internal carotid artery and carotid plexus

Nerve to stylo-pharyngeus
Communication with branch of facial to stylo-
hyoid and posterior belly of digastric
Lingual branch (of facial)

Nerves to pharyngeal plexus
Mucous membrane of tonsil
Palato-glossal arch

tongue

Lingual branches

Tonsillar plexus

PLATE 157.—VAGUS NERVE

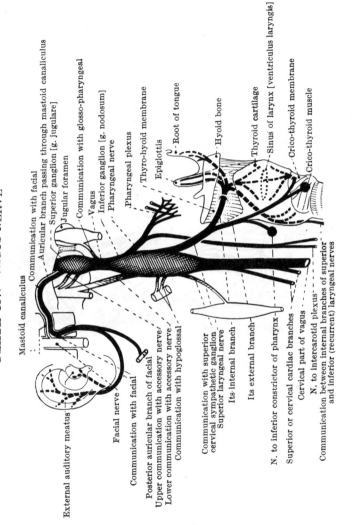

Mastoid canaliculus
Communication with facial
Auricular branch passing through mastoid canaliculus
Superior ganglion [g. jugulare]
Jugular foramen
Communication with glosso-pharyngeal
Vagus
Inferior ganglion [g. nodosum]
Pharyngeal nerve
Pharyngeal plexus
Thyro-hyoid membrane
Epiglottis
Root of tongue
Hyoid bone
Thyroid cartilage
Sinus of larynx [ventriculus laryngis]
Crico-thyroid membrane
Crico-thyroid muscle

External auditory meatus

Facial nerve

Communication with facial
Posterior auricular branch of facial
Upper communication with accessory nerve
Lower communication with accessory nerve
Communication with hypoglossal

Communication with superior
cervical sympathetic ganglion
Superior laryngeal nerve
Its internal branch

Its external branch

N. to inferior constrictor of pharynx
Superior or cervical cardiac branches
Cervical part of vagus
N. to intercarotid plexus
Communication between internal branches of superior
and inferior (recurrent) laryngeal nerves

PLATE 158.—VAGUS NERVE (*Continued*)

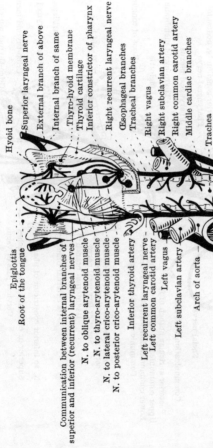

Epiglottis
Root of the tongue
Hyoid bone
Superior laryngeal nerve
External branch of above
Internal branch of same
Thyro-hyoid membrane
Thyroid cartilage
Inferior constrictor of pharynx
Right recurrent laryngeal nerve
Œsophageal branches
Tracheal branches
Right vagus
Right subclavian artery
Right common carotid artery
Middle cardiac branches
Trachea
Lower cardiac branches
Right pulmonary plexus, surrounding right bronchus

Communication between internal branches of superior and inferior (recurrent) laryngeal nerves
N. to oblique arytenoid muscle
N. to thyro-arytenoid muscle
N. to lateral crico-arytenoid muscle
N. to posterior crico-arytenoid muscle
Inferior thyroid artery
Left recurrent laryngeal nerve
Left common carotid artery
Left vagus
Left subclavian artery
Arch of aorta
Inferior cardiac branches
Left pulmonary plexus surrounding left bronchus

PLATE 159.—VAGUS NERVE (*Continued*)

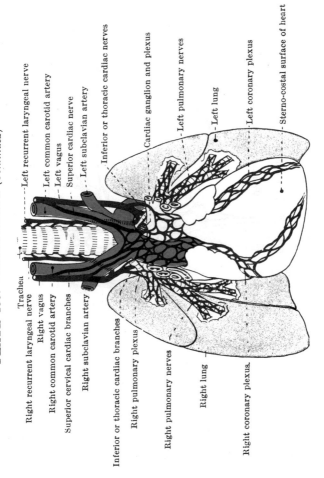

PLATE 160.—VAGUS NERVE (Continued)

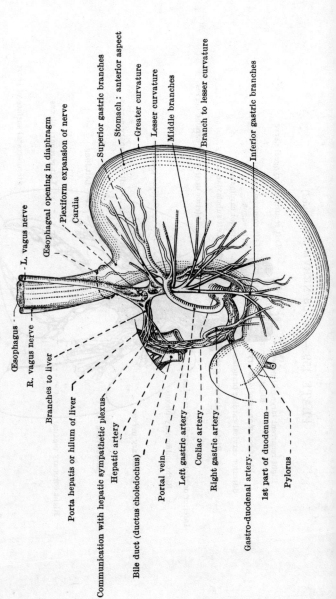

PLATE 161.—VAGUS NERVE (*Continued*)

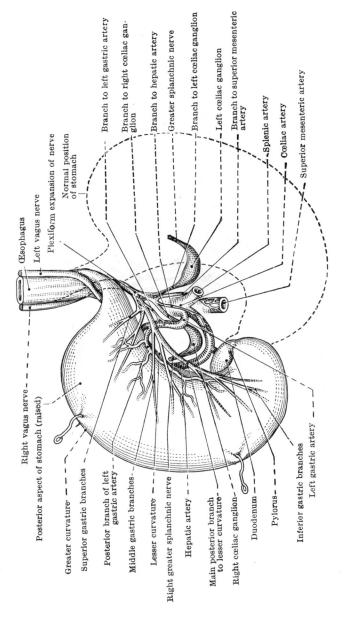

Right vagus nerve
Posterior aspect of stomach (raised)

Œsophagus
Left vagus nerve
Plexiform expansion of nerve
Normal position of stomach

Branch to left gastric artery
Branch to right cœliac gan-glion
Branch to hepatic artery
Greater splanchnic nerve
Branch to left cœliac ganglion
Left cœliac ganglion
Branch to superior mesenteric artery
Splenic artery
Cœliac artery
Superior mesenteric artery

Greater curvature
Superior gastric branches
Posterior branch of left gastric artery
Middle gastric branches
Lesser curvature
Hepatic artery
Right greater splanchnic nerve
Main posterior branch to lesser curvature
Right cœliac ganglion
Duodenum
Pylorus
Inferior gastric branches
Left gastric artery

11

PLATE 162.—ACCESSORY NERVE

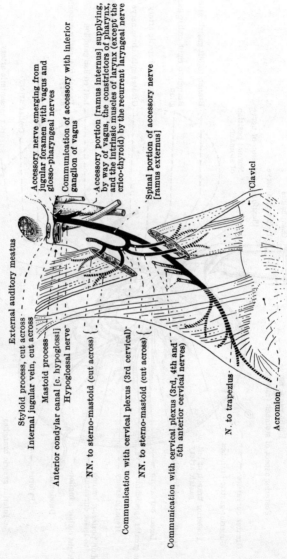

External auditory meatus

Accessory nerve emerging from jugular foramen with vagus and glosso-pharyngeal nerves

Communication of accessory with inferior ganglion of vagus

Accessory portion [ramus internus] supplying, by way of vagus, the constrictors of pharynx, and the intrinsic muscles of larynx (except the crico-thyroid) by the recurrent laryngeal nerve

Spinal portion of accessory nerve [ramus externus]

Styloid process, cut across
Internal jugular vein, cut across
Mastoid process
Anterior condylar canal [c. hypoglossi]
Hypoglossal nerve

NN. to sterno-mastoid (cut across) {

Communication with cervical plexus (3rd cervical)

NN. to sterno-mastoid (cut across) {

Communication with cervical plexus (3rd, 4th and 5th anterior cervical nerves)

N. to trapezius

Acromion

Clavicl

PLATE 163.—HYPOGLOSSAL NERVE

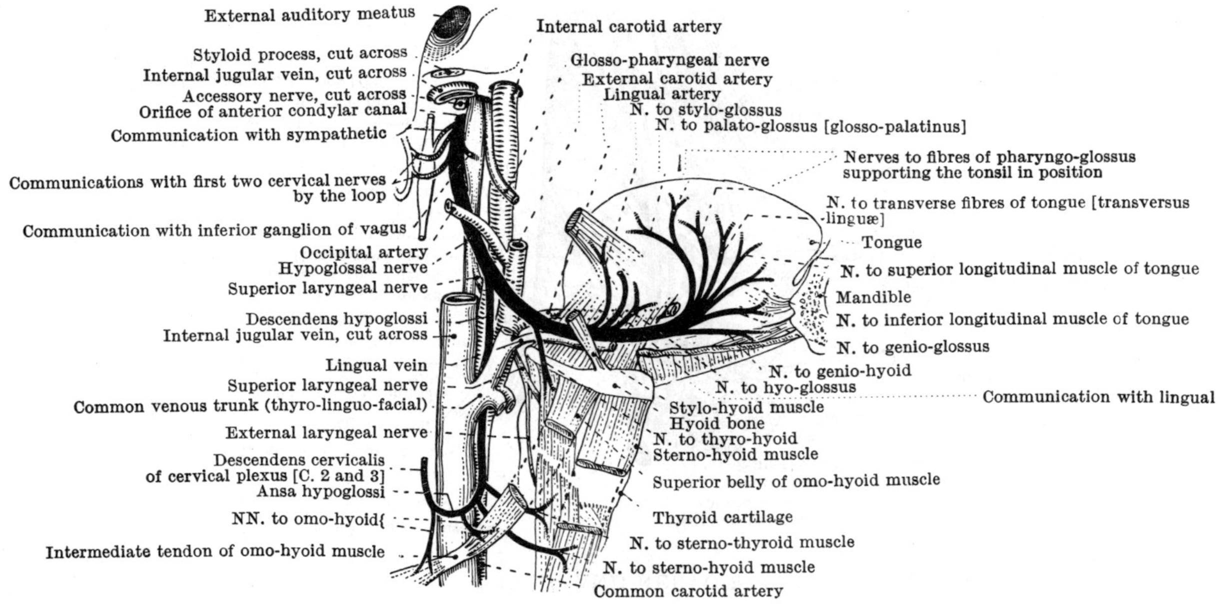

External auditory meatus

Styloid process, cut across
Internal jugular vein, cut across
Accessory nerve, cut across
Orifice of anterior condylar canal
Communication with sympathetic

Communications with first two cervical nerves
by the loop

Communication with inferior ganglion of vagus
Occipital artery
Hypoglossal nerve
Superior laryngeal nerve

Descendens hypoglossi
Internal jugular vein, cut across
Lingual vein
Superior laryngeal nerve
Common venous trunk (thyro-linguo-facial)
External laryngeal nerve
Descendens cervicalis
of cervical plexus [C. 2 and 3]
Ansa hypoglossi

NN. to omo-hyoid

Intermediate tendon of omo-hyoid muscle

Internal carotid artery

Glosso-pharyngeal nerve
External carotid artery
Lingual artery
N. to stylo-glossus
N. to palato-glossus [glosso-palatinus]

Nerves to fibres of pharyngo-glossus
supporting the tonsil in position

N. to transverse fibres of tongue [transversus
linguæ]

Tongue

N. to superior longitudinal muscle of tongue
Mandible
N. to inferior longitudinal muscle of tongue
N. to genio-glossus

Communication with lingual

N. to genio-hyoid
N. to hyo-glossus
Stylo-hyoid muscle
Hyoid bone
N. to thyro-hyoid
Sterno-hyoid muscle
Superior belly of omo-hyoid muscle
Thyroid cartilage
N. to sterno-thyroid muscle
N. to sterno-hyoid muscle
Common carotid artery

PLATE 164.—VASCULAR AND NERVOUS RELATIONS IN NECK

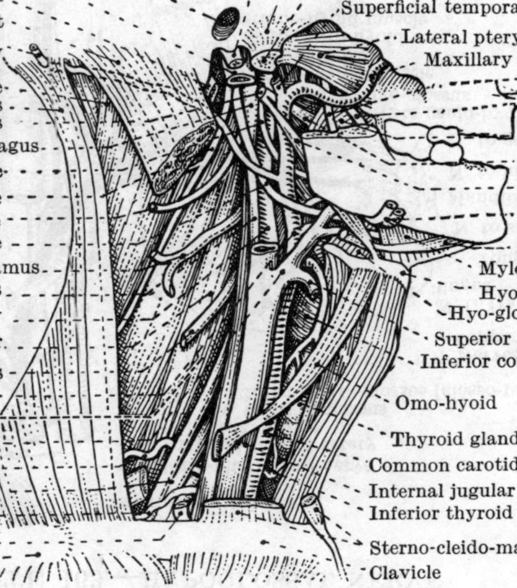

External auditory meatus

Internal jugular vein, cut
Digastric muscle, cut
Sterno-cleido-mastoid, cut
Occipital artery
Splenius capitis muscle
Trapezius
Styloid process, cut across
Inferior ganglion of vagus
Glosso-pharyngeal nerve
Accessory nerve
Lesser occipital nerve
Hypoglossal nerve
3rd cervical nerve, anterior ramus
Vagus
Internal carotid artery
Scalenus posterior
4th cervical nerve, anterior ramus
External carotid artery
Scalenus medius
Thyro-linguo-facial venous trunk
Transverse cervical artery
Brachial plexus
Suprascapular artery
External jugular vein, cut across
Acromion

Styloid process, cut across
Mandibular joint
Neck of mandible, cut across
Superficial temporal artery, cut
Lateral pterygoid muscle
Maxillary artery
Inferior dental nerve
Lingual nerve
Medial pterygoid muscle
Stylo-glossus
Facial [a. maxillaris external]
artery and vein
Anterior belly of digastric
Mylo-hyoid
Hyoid bone
Stylo-hyoid
Hyo-glossus
Superior thyroid artery and vein
Inferior constrictor of pharynx
Omo-hyoid
Thyroid gland, right lobe
Common carotid artery
Internal jugular vein
Inferior thyroid artery
Sterno-cleido-mastoid, cut across
Clavicle

PLATE 165.—CERVICAL SYMPATHETIC NERVES
(AFTER HOVELACQUE)

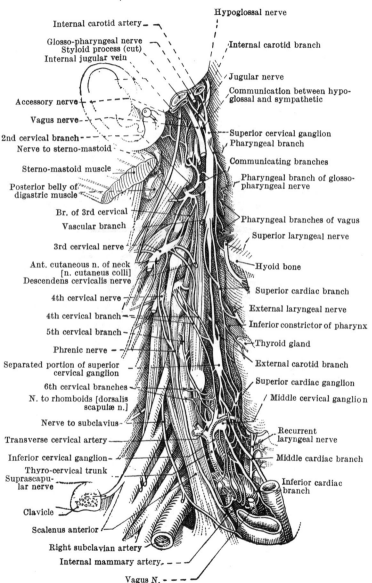

Hypoglossal nerve

Internal carotid artery

Glosso-pharyngeal nerve
Styloid process (cut)
Internal jugular vein

Internal carotid branch

Jugular nerve

Communication between hypoglossal and sympathetic

Accessory nerve

Vagus nerve

2nd cervical branch
Nerve to sterno-mastoid

Superior cervical ganglion
Pharyngeal branch

Communicating branches

Sterno-mastoid muscle

Posterior belly of
digastric muscle

Pharyngeal branch of glosso-
pharyngeal nerve

Br. of 3rd cervical
Vascular branch

Pharyngeal branches of vagus

Superior laryngeal nerve

3rd cervical nerve

Ant. cutaneous n. of neck
[n. cutaneus colli]
Descendens cervicalis nerve

Hyoid bone

4th cervical nerve

Superior cardiac branch

4th cervical branch

External laryngeal nerve

5th cervical branch

Inferior constrictor of pharynx

Phrenic nerve

Thyroid gland

Separated portion of superior
cervical ganglion

External carotid branch

6th cervical branches

Superior cardiac ganglion

N. to rhomboids [dorsalis
scapulæ n.]

Middle cervical ganglion

Nerve to subclavius

Recurrent
laryngeal nerve

Transverse cervical artery

Inferior cervical ganglion

Middle cardiac branch

Thyro-cervical trunk
Suprascapu-
lar nerve

Inferior cardiac
branch

Clavicle

Scalenus anterior

Right subclavian artery

Internal mammary artery

Vagus N.

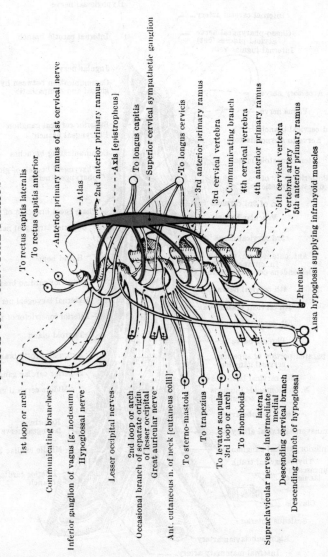

PLATE 166.—CERVICAL PLEXUS

1st loop or arch
Communicating branches
Inferior ganglion of vagus [g. nodosum]
Hypoglossal nerve
Lesser occipital nerves
2nd loop or arch
Occasional branch of separate origin of lesser occipital
Great auricular nerve
Ant. cutaneous n. of neck [cutaneus colli]
Supraclavicular nerves { lateral { intermediate { medial
Descending cervical branch
Descending branch of hypoglossal

To rectus capitis lateralis
To rectus capitis anterior
Anterior primary ramus of 1st cervical nerve
Atlas
2nd anterior primary ramus
Axis [epistropheus]
To longus capitis
Superior cervical sympathetic ganglion
To longus cervicis
3rd anterior primary ramus
3rd cervical vertebra
Communicating branch
4th cervical vertebra
4th anterior primary ramus
5th cervical vertebra
Vertebral artery
5th anterior primary ramus
Phrenic
Ansa hypoglossi supplying infrahyoid muscles

To sterno-mastoid
To trapezius
To levator scapulæ
3rd loop or arch
To rhomboids

PLATE 167.—CERVICAL PLEXUS—PHRENIC NERVE AND BRANCHES

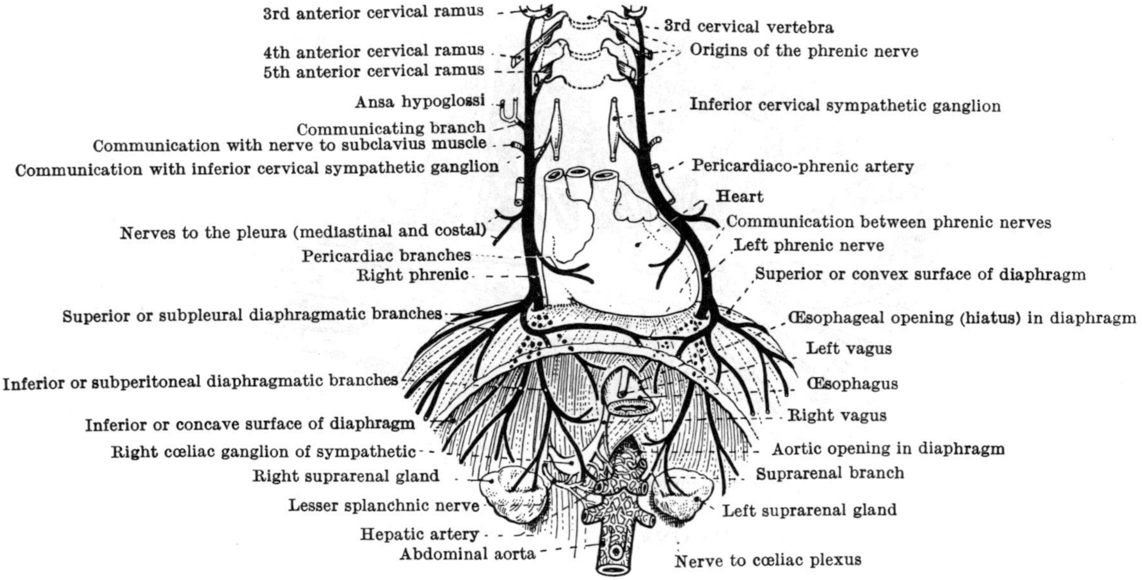

3rd anterior cervical ramus
3rd cervical vertebra
Origins of the phrenic nerve
4th anterior cervical ramus
5th anterior cervical ramus
Inferior cervical sympathetic ganglion
Ansa hypoglossi
Communicating branch
Communication with nerve to subclavius muscle
Communication with inferior cervical sympathetic ganglion
Pericardiaco-phrenic artery
Heart
Communication between phrenic nerves
Left phrenic nerve
Superior or convex surface of diaphragm
Nerves to the pleura (mediastinal and costal)
Pericardiac branches
Right phrenic
Oesophageal opening (hiatus) in diaphragm
Left vagus
Oesophagus
Right vagus
Superior or subpleural diaphragmatic branches
Aortic opening in diaphragm
Suprarenal branch
Left suprarenal gland
Inferior or subperitoneal diaphragmatic branches
Inferior or concave surface of diaphragm
Right ceeliac ganglion of sympathetic
Right suprarenal gland
Lesser splanchnic nerve
Nerve to celiac plexus
Hepatic artery
Abdominal aorta

PLATE 168.—AXILLA AND ITS CONTENTS

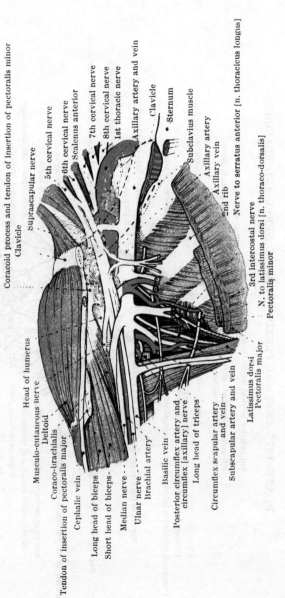

Coracoid process and tendon of insertion of pectoralis minor
Clavicle
Suprascapular nerve
5th cervical nerve
6th cervical nerve
Scalenus anterior
7th cervical nerve
8th cervical nerve
1st thoracic nerve
Axillary artery and vein
Clavicle
Sternum
Subclavius muscle
Axillary artery
Axillary vein
2nd rib
Nerve to serratus anterior [n. thoracicus longus]
3rd intercostal nerve
N. to latissimus dorsi [n. thoraco-dorsalis]
Pectoralis minor
Latissimus dorsi
Pectoralis major
Subscapular artery and vein
Circumflex scapular artery and vein
Long head of triceps
Posterior circumflex artery and circumflex [axillary] nerve
Basilic vein
Brachial artery
Ulnar nerve
Median nerve
Short head of biceps
Long head of biceps
Cephalic vein
Tendon of insertion of pectoralis major
Coraco-brachialis
Deltoid
Musculo-cutaneous nerve
Head of humerus

PLATE 169.—DIAGRAM OF BRACHIAL PLEXUS

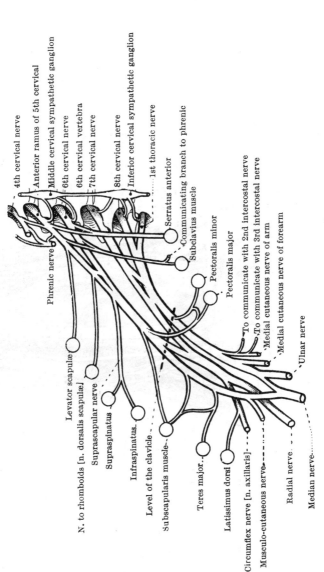

PLATE 170.—PHARYNX AND ITS RELATIONS

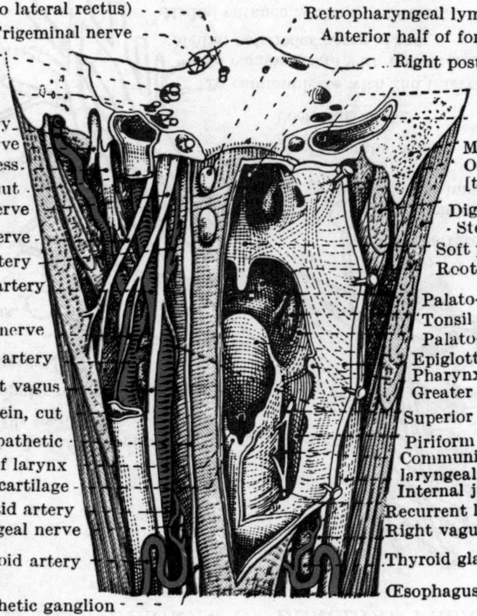

Abducent nerve (to lateral rectus)
Trigeminal nerve
Facial and auditory nerves
Glosso-pharyngeal, vagus, and accessory nerves
Occipital artery
Facial nerve
Styloid process
Internal jugular vein, cut
Hypoglossal nerve
Accessory nerve
Ascending pharyngeal artery
Internal carotid artery
Descending branch of hypoglossal nerve
External carotid artery
Left vagus
Internal jugular vein, cut
Cervical sympathetic
Cavity of larynx
Left arytenoid cartilage
Common carotid artery
Left recurrent laryngeal nerve
Inferior thyroid artery
Middle cervical sympathetic ganglion

Retropharyngeal lymph glands
Anterior half of foramen magnum
Right posterior aperture of nose [choana]
Internal jugular vein
Sigmoid sinus
Mastoid process
Opening of the pharyngo-tympanic tube [tuba auditiva]
Digastric muscle, cut
Sterno-cleido-mastoid
Soft palate
Root of tongue
Palato-glossal arch
Tonsil
Palato-pharyngeal arch
Epiglottis
Pharynx
Greater horn of hyoid bone
Superior laryngeal nerves
Piriform fossa
Communication between superior and recurrent laryngeal nerves
Internal jugular vein
Recurrent laryngeal nerve
Right vagus
Thyroid gland
Œsophagus

PLATE 171.—HORIZONTAL SECTION AT THE LEVEL OF THE CLAVICLES

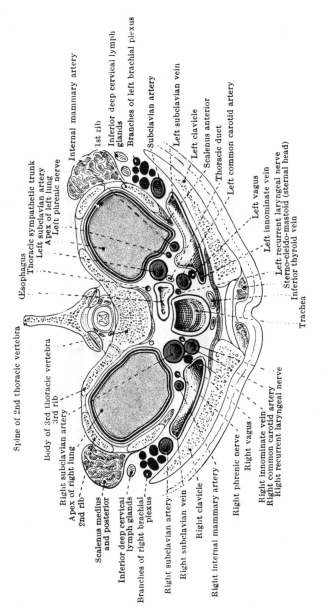

Spine of 2nd thoracic vertebra

Œsophagus
Thoracic sympathetic trunk
Left subclavian artery
Apex of left lung
Left phrenic nerve

Internal mammary artery

1st rib
Inferior deep cervical lymph glands
Branches of left brachial plexus

Subclavian artery

Left subclavian vein

Left clavicle

Scalenus anterior

Thoracic duct

Left common carotid artery

Left vagus

Left innominate vein

Left recurrent laryngeal nerve
Sterno-cleido-mastoid (sternal head)
Inferior thyroid vein

Trachea

Body of 3rd thoracic vertebra
3rd rib

Right subclavian artery
Apex of right lung
2nd rib

Scalenus medius
and posterior

Inferior deep cervical
lymph glands

Branches of right brachial
plexus

Right subclavian artery

Right subclavian vein

Right clavicle

Right internal mammary artery

Right phrenic nerve

Right vagus

Right innominate vein
Right common carotid artery
Right recurrent laryngeal nerve

PLATE 172.—ANTERIOR MUSCLES OF TRUNK

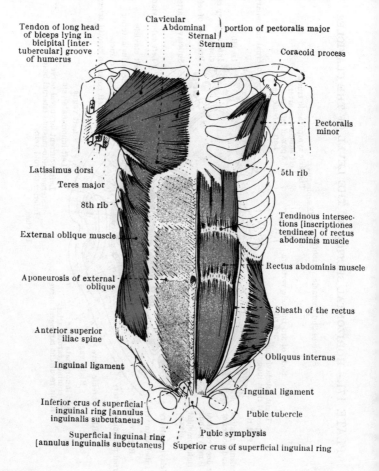

Tendon of long head of biceps lying in bicipital [inter-tubercular] groove of humerus

Clavicular
Abdominal } portion of pectoralis major
Sternal
Sternum

Coracoid process

Pectoralis minor

Latissimus dorsi

Teres major

8th rib

External oblique muscle

5th rib

Tendinous intersections [inscriptiones tendineæ] of rectus abdominis muscle

Rectus abdominis muscle

Aponeurosis of external oblique

Sheath of the rectus

Anterior superior iliac spine

Obliquus internus

Inguinal ligament

Inguinal ligament

Inferior crus of superficial inguinal ring [annulus inguinalis subcutaneus]

Pubic tubercle

Superficial inguinal ring [annulus inguinalis subcutaneus]

Pubic symphysis

Superior crus of superficial inguinal ring

PLATE 173

INTERNAL MAMMARY AND EPIGASTRIC ARTERIES

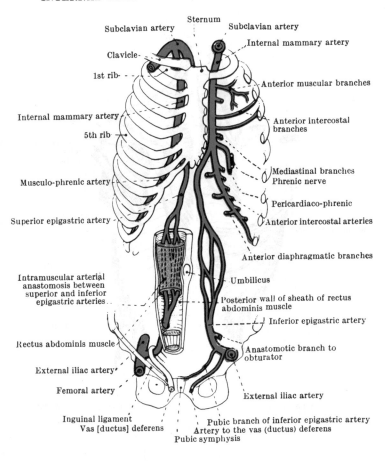

Sternum

Subclavian artery

Subclavian artery

Internal mammary artery

Clavicle

Anterior muscular branches

1st rib

Internal mammary artery

Anterior intercostal branches

5th rib

Mediastinal branches
Phrenic nerve

Musculo-phrenic artery

Pericardiaco-phrenic

Superior epigastric artery

Anterior intercostal arteries

Anterior diaphragmatic branches

Intramuscular arterial anastomosis between superior and inferior epigastric arteries

Umbilicus

Posterior wall of sheath of rectus abdominis muscle

Inferior epigastric artery

Rectus abdominis muscle

Anastomotic branch to obturator

External iliac artery

Femoral artery

External iliac artery

Inguinal ligament
Vas [ductus] deferens

Pubic branch of inferior epigastric artery
Artery to the vas (ductus) deferens
Pubic symphysis

PLATE 174.—POSTERIOR MUSCLES OF TRUNK

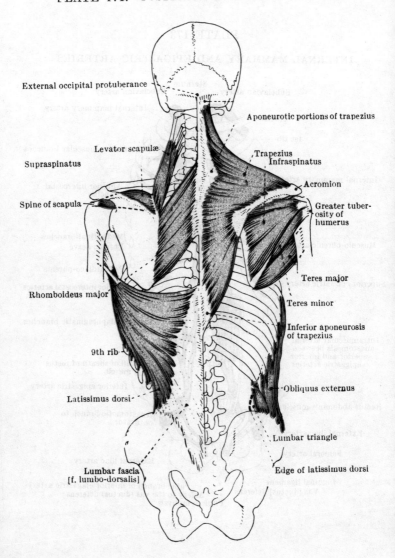

External occipital protuberance

Aponeurotic portions of trapezius

Levator scapulæ

Trapezius
Infraspinatus

Supraspinatus

Acromion

Spine of scapula

Greater tuberosity of humerus

Teres major

Teres minor

Rhomboideus major

Inferior aponeurosis of trapezius

9th rib

Latissimus dorsi

Obliquus externus

Lumbar triangle

Lumbar fascia
[f. lumbo-dorsalis]

Edge of latissimus dorsi

PLATE 175.—POSTERIOR VERTEBRAL MUSCLES

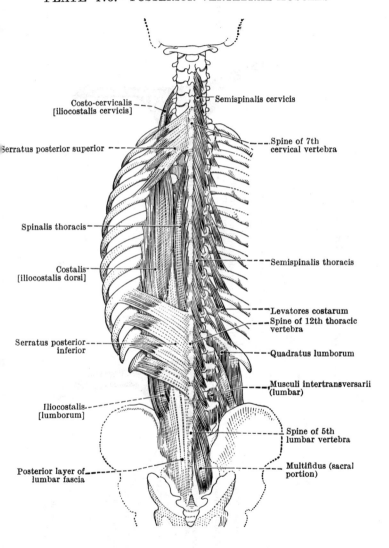

Costo-cervicalis [iliocostalis cervicis]

Semispinalis cervicis

Serratus posterior superior

Spine of 7th cervical vertebra

Spinalis thoracis

Costalis [iliocostalis dorsi]

Semispinalis thoracis

Levatores costarum

Spine of 12th thoracic vertebra

Serratus posterior inferior

Quadratus lumborum

Musculi intertransversarii (lumbar)

Iliocostalis [lumborum]

Spine of 5th lumbar vertebra

Posterior layer of lumbar fascia

Multifidus (sacral portion)

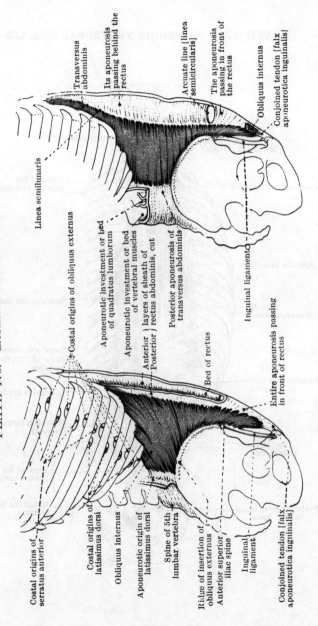

PLATE 176.—LATERAL TRUNK MUSCLES

Transversus abdominis

Its aponeurosis passing behind the rectus

Arcuate line [linea semicircularis]

The aponeurosis passing in front of the rectus

Obliquus internus

Conjoined tendon [falx aponeurotica inguinalis]

Linea semilunaris

Costal origins of obliquus externus

Aponeurotic investment or bed of quadratus lumborum

Aponeurotic investment or bed of vertebral muscles

Anterior } layers of sheath of
Posterior } rectus abdominis, cut

Posterior aponeurosis of transversus abdominis

Bed of rectus

Inguinal ligament

Entire aponeurosis passing in front of rectus

Costal origins of serratus anterior

Costal origins of latissimus dorsi

Obliquus internus

Aponeurotic origin of latissimus dorsi

Spine of 5th lumbar vertebra

Ridge of insertion of obliquus externus

Anterior superior iliac spine

Inguinal ligament

Conjoined tendon [falx aponeurotica inguinalis]

PLATE 177.—INGUINAL CANAL

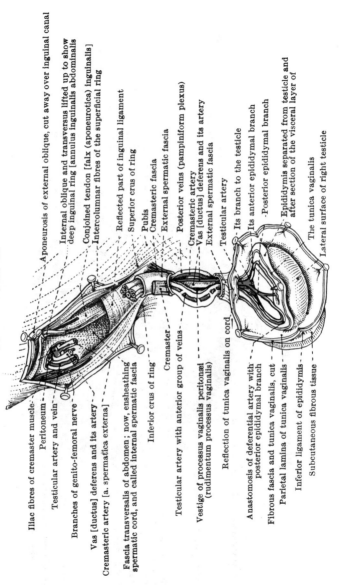

Inferior epigastric artery and vein

Illac fibres of cremaster muscle
Peritoneum
Testicular artery and vein
Branches of genito-femoral nerve
Vas [ductus] deferens and its artery
Cremasteric artery [a. spermafica externa]

Fascia transversalis of abdomen; now, ensheathing spermatic cord, and called internal spermatic fascia

Inferior crus of ring

Cremaster

Testicular artery with anterior group of veins

Vestige of processus vaginalis peritonei (rudimentum processus vaginalis)

Reflection of tunica vaginalis on cord

Anastomosis of deferential artery with posterior epididymal branch
Fibrous fascia and tunica vaginalis, cut
Parietal lamina of tunica vaginalis
Inferior ligament of epididymis
Subcutaneous fibrous tissue

Aponeurosis of external oblique, cut away over inguinal canal
Internal oblique and transversus lifted up to show deep inguinal ring [annulus inguinalis abdominalis]
Conjoined tendon [falx (aponeurotica) inguinalis]
Intercolumnar fibres of the superficial ring

Reflected part of inguinal ligament
Superior crus of ring
Pubis
Cremasteric fascia
External spermatic fascia

Posterior veins (pampiniform plexus)

Cremasteric artery
Vas [ductus] deferens and its artery
External spermatic fascia

Testicular artery

Its branch to the testicle
Its anterior epididymal branch
Posterior epididymal branch

Epididymis separated from testicle and after section of the visceral layer of

The tunica vaginalis
Lateral surface of right testicle

12

PLATE 178.—DIAPHRAGM (INFERIOR ASPECT)

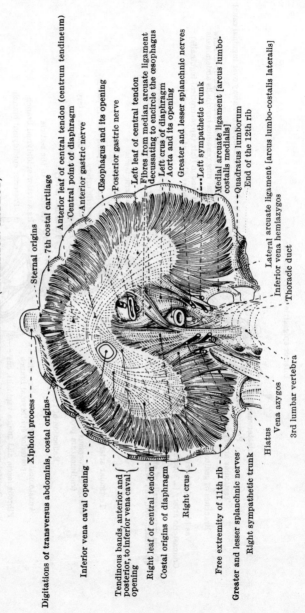

Xiphoid process

Sternal origins

Digitations of transversus abdominis, costal origins

7th costal cartilage

Anterior leaf of central tendon (centrum tendineum)

Central point of diaphragm

Anterior gastric nerve

Œsophagus and its opening

Posterior gastric nerve

Left leaf of central tendon

Fibres from median arcuate ligament decussating to encircle the œsophagus

Left crus of diaphragm

Aorta and its opening

Greater and lesser splanchnic nerves

Left sympathetic trunk

Medial arcuate ligament [arcus lumbo-costalis medialis]

Quadratus lumborum

End of the 12th rib

Lateral arcuate ligament [arcus lumbo-costalis lateralis]

Inferior vena hemiazygos

Thoracic duct

Inferior vena caval opening

Tendinous bands, anterior and posterior, to inferior vena caval opening

Right leaf of central tendon

Costal origins of diaphragm

Right crus

Free extremity of 11th rib

Greater and lesser splanchnic nerves

Right sympathetic trunk

Hiatus

Vena azygos

3rd lumbar vertebra

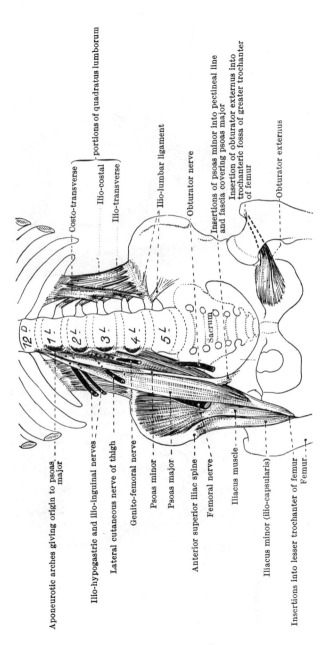

PLATE 179.—MUSCLES OF POSTERIOR WALL OF ABDOMEN

Aponeurotic arches giving origin to psoas major

Ilio-hypogastric and ilio-inguinal nerves

Lateral cutaneous nerve of thigh

Genito-femoral nerve

Psoas minor

Psoas major

Anterior superior iliac spine

Femoral nerve

Iliacus muscle

Iliacus minor (ilio-capsularis)

Insertions into lesser trochanter of femur
Femur

Costo-transverse
Ilio-costal } portions of quadratus lumborum
Ilio-transverse

Ilio-lumbar ligament

Obturator nerve

Insertions of psoas minor into pectineal line and fascia covering psoas major

Insertion of obturator externus into trochanteric fossa of greater trochanter of femur

Obturator externus

Sacrum

PLATE 180.—MEDIAL SURFACE OF LUNGS

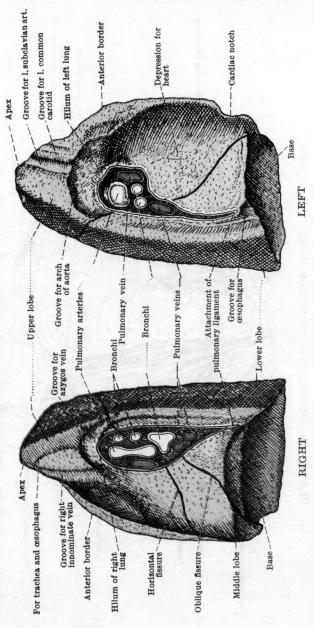

Apex — Groove for l. subclavian art. — Groove for l. common carotid — Hilum of left lung — Anterior border — Depression for heart — Cardiac notch — Base — **LEFT**

Upper lobe — Groove for arch of aorta — Pulmonary arteries — Bronchi — Pulmonary vein — Bronchi — Pulmonary veins — Attachment of pulmonary ligament — Groove for œsophagus — Lower lobe — Groove for azygos vein

Apex — For trachea and œsophagus — Groove for right innominate vein — Anterior border — Hilum of right lung — Horizontal fissure — Oblique fissure — Middle lobe — Base — **RIGHT**

PLATE 181.—RELATIONS OF LUNGS TO THORACIC WALL

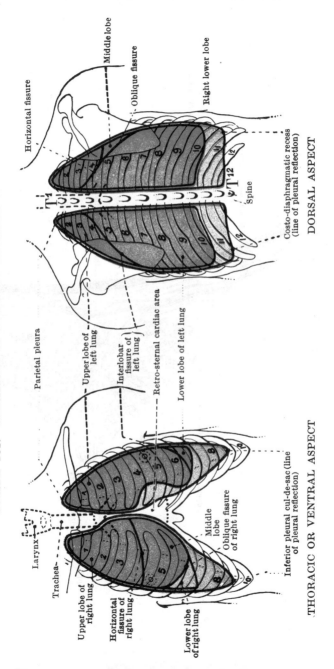

Horizontal fissure

Middle lobe

Oblique fissure

Right lower lobe

Costo-diaphragmatic recess (line of pleural reflection)

Spine

T 12

DORSAL ASPECT

Parietal pleura

Upper lobe of left lung

Interlobar fissure of left lung

Retro-sternal cardiac area

Lower lobe of left lung

Larynx

Trachea

Upper lobe of right lung

Horizontal fissure of right lung

Lower lobe of right lung

Middle lobe

Oblique fissure of right lung

Inferior pleural cul-de-sac (line of pleural reflection)

THORACIC OR VENTRAL ASPECT

PLATE 182.—VERTICAL SECTION OF MAMMARY GLAND

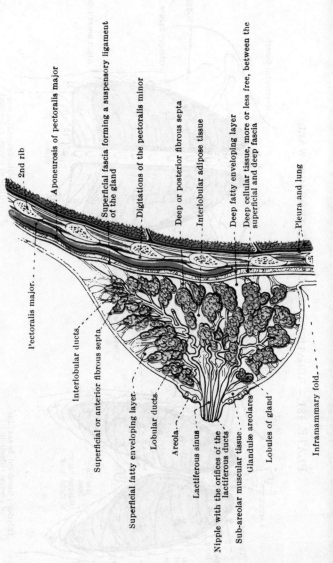

2nd rib

Aponeurosis of pectoralis major

Superficial fascia forming a suspensory ligament of the gland

Digitations of the pectoralis minor

Deep or posterior fibrous septa

Interlobular adipose tissue

Deep fatty enveloping layer

Deep cellular tissue, more or less free, between the superficial and deep fascia

Pleura and lung

Pectoralis major

Interlobular ducts

Superficial or anterior fibrous septa

Superficial fatty enveloping layer

Lobular ducts

Areola

Lactiferous sinus

Nipple with the orifices of the lactiferous ducts

Sub-areolar muscular tissue

Glandulæ areolares

Lobules of gland

Inframammary fold

PLATE 183.—LYMPHATICS OF THE BREAST

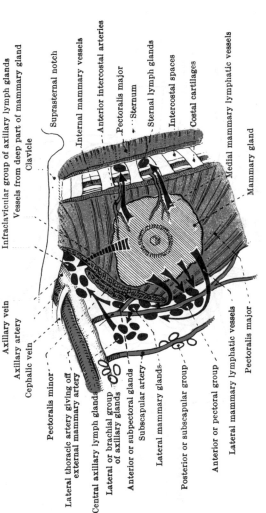

Infraclavicular group of axillary lymph glands
Vessels from deep part of mammary gland
Clavicle
Suprasternal notch
Internal mammary vessels
Anterior intercostal arteries
Pectoralis major
Sternum
Sternal lymph glands
Intercostal spaces
Costal cartilages
Medial mammary lymphatic vessels
Mammary gland
Pectoralis major
Lateral mammary lymphatic vessels
Anterior or pectoral group
Posterior or subscapular group
Lateral mammary glands
Subscapular artery
Anterior or subpectoral glands
Lateral or brachial group of axillary glands
Central axillary lymph glands
Lateral thoracic artery giving off external mammary artery
Pectoralis minor
Cephalic vein
Axillary artery
Axillary vein

Note.—The breast tissue is more extensive than shown.

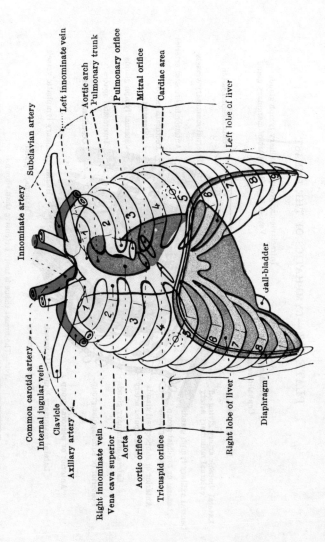

PLATE 184.—RELATIONS OF HEART TO THORACIC WALL

Common carotid artery
Internal jugular vein
Clavicle
Axillary artery

Right innominate vein
Vena cava superior
Aorta
Aortic orifice
Tricuspid orifice

Right lobe of liver

Diaphragm

Innominate artery

Subclavian artery

Left innominate vein
Aortic arch
Pulmonary trunk

Pulmonary orifice

Mitral orifice

Cardiac area

Left lobe of liver

Gall-bladder

PLATE 185.—CONTENTS OF MEDIASTINUM—ANTERIOR ASPECT

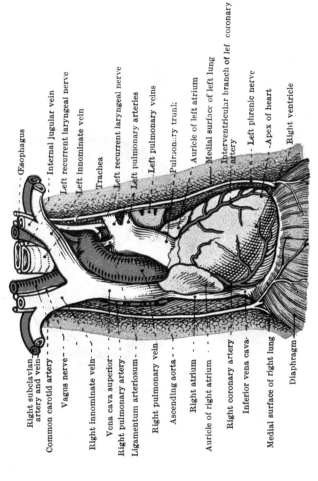

Œsophagus

Internal jugular vein

Left recurrent laryngeal nerve

Left innominate vein

Trachea

Left recurrent laryngeal nerve

Left pulmonary arteries

Left pulmonary veins

Pulmonary trunk

Auricle of left atrium

Medial surface of left lung

Interventricular branch of lef coronary artery

Left phrenic nerve

Apex of heart

Right ventricle

Right subclavian artery and vein

Common carotid artery

Vagus nerve

Right innominate vein

Vena cava superior

Right pulmonary artery

Ligamentum arteriosum

Right pulmonary vein

Ascending aorta

Right atrium

Auricle of right atrium

Right coronary artery

Inferior vena cava

Medial surface of right lung

Diaphragm

PLATE 186.—HEART—STERNO-COSTAL SURFACE

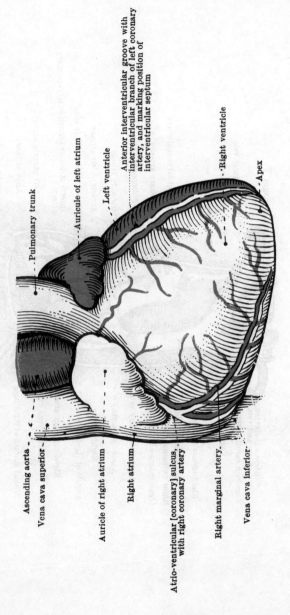

Pulmonary trunk

Auricule of left atrium

Left ventricle

Anterior interventricular groove with
interventricular branch of left coronary
artery, and marking position of
interventricular septum

Right ventricle

Apex

Ascending aorta

Vena cava superior

Auricle of right atrium

Right atrium

Atrio-ventricular [coronary] sulcus,
with right coronary artery

Right marginal artery

Vena cava inferior

PLATE 187.—HEART—CORONAL SECTION

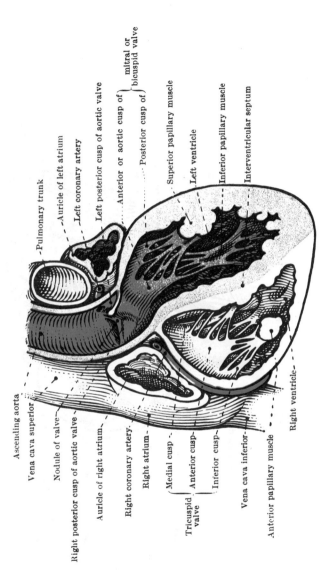

Ascending aorta
Vena cava superior
Nodule of valve
Right posterior cusp of aortic valve
Auricle of right atrium
Right coronary artery
Right atrium
Medial cusp
Anterior cusp
Tricuspid valve
Inferior cusp
Vena cava inferior
Anterior papillary muscle
Right ventricle

Pulmonary trunk
Auricle of left atrium
Left coronary artery
Left posterior cusp of aortic valve
Anterior or aortic cusp of mitral or bicuspid valve
Posterior cusp of
Superior papillary muscle
Left ventricle
Inferior papillary muscle
Interventricular septum

PLATE 188.—RIGHT SIDE OF HEART, CUT OPEN

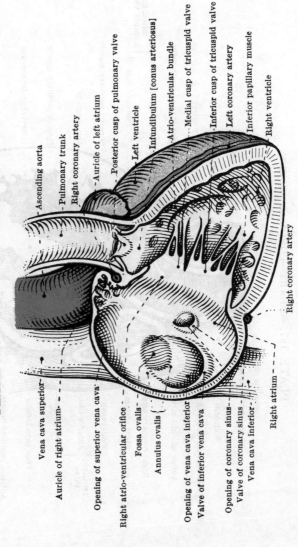

Vena cava superior

Auricle of right atrium

Opening of superior vena cava

Right atrio-ventricular orifice

Fossa ovalis

Annulus ovalis

Opening of vena cava inferior

Valve of inferior vena cava

Opening of coronary sinus

Valve of coronary sinus

Vena cava inferior

Right atrium

Ascending aorta

Pulmonary trunk

Right coronary artery

Auricle of left atrium

Posterior cusp of pulmonary valve

Left ventricle

Infundibulum [conus arteriosus]

Atrio-ventricular bundle

Medial cusp of tricuspid valve

Inferior cusp of tricuspid valve

Left coronary artery

Inferior papillary muscle

Right ventricle

Right coronary artery

PLATE 189.—DIAGRAM OF THE CIRCULATION

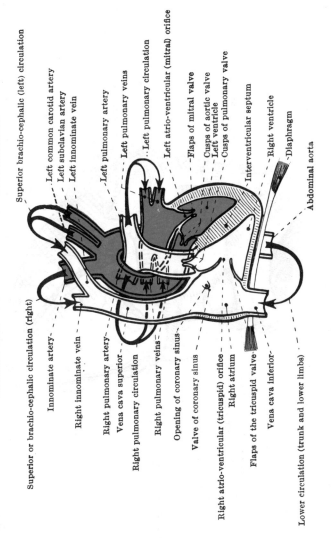

Superior or brachio-cephalic circulation (right)

Superior brachio-cephalic (left) circulation

Left common carotid artery

Left subclavian artery

Left innominate vein

Left pulmonary artery

Left pulmonary veins

Left pulmonary circulation

Left atrio-ventricular (mitral) orifice

Flaps of mitral valve

Cusps of aortic valve

Left ventricle

Cusps of pulmonary valve

Interventricular septum

Right ventricle

Diaphragm

Abdominal aorta

Innominate artery

Right innominate vein

Right pulmonary artery

Vena cava superior

Right pulmonary circulation

Right pulmonary veins

Opening of coronary sinus

Valve of coronary sinus

Right atrium

Right atrio-ventricular (tricuspid) orifice

Flaps of the tricuspid valve

Vena cava inferior

Lower circulation (trunk and lower limbs)

PLATE 190.—HEART—POSTERIOR ASPECT

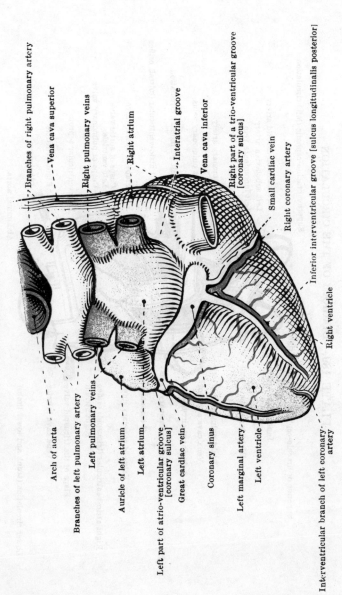

Branches of right pulmonary artery
Vena cava superior
Right pulmonary veins
Right atrium
Interatrial groove
Vena cava inferior
Right part of a trio-ventricular groove [coronary sulcus]
Small cardiac vein
Right coronary artery
Inferior interventricular groove [sulcus longitudinalis posterior]
Right ventricle

Arch of aorta
Branches of left pulmonary artery
Left pulmonary veins
Auricle of left atrium
Left atrium
Left part of atrio-ventricular groove [coronary sulcus]
Great cardiac vein
Coronary sinus
Left marginal artery
Left ventricle
Interventricular branch of left coronary artery

PLATE 191.—LEFT SIDE OF HEART, CUT OPEN

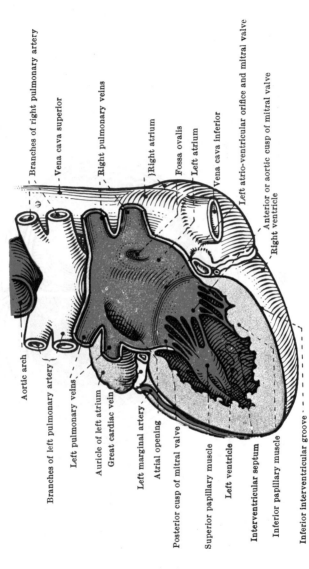

Aortic arch

Branches of left pulmonary artery

Left pulmonary veins

Auricle of left atrium

Great cardiac vein

Left marginal artery

Atrial opening

Posterior cusp of mitral valve

Superior papillary muscle

Left ventricle

Interventricular septum

Inferior papillary muscle

Inferior interventricular groove

Branches of right pulmonary artery

Vena cava superior

Right pulmonary veins

Right atrium

Fossa ovalis

Left atrium

Vena cava inferior

Left atrio-ventricular orifice and mitral valve

Anterior or aortic cusp of mitral valve

Right ventricle

PLATE 192.—BASE OF VENTRICLES, SHOWING ORIFICES AND VALVES

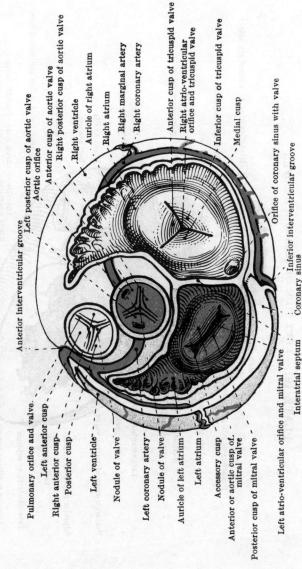

Anterior interventricular groove

Left posterior cusp of aortic valve
Aortic orifice
Anterior cusp of aortic valve
Right posterior cusp of aortic valve
Right ventricle
Auricle of right atrium
Right atrium
Right marginal artery
Right coronary artery
Anterior cusp of tricuspid valve
Right atrio-ventricular orifice and tricuspid valve
Inferior cusp of tricuspid valve
Medial cusp
Orifice of coronary sinus with valve
Inferior interventricular groove
Coronary sinus

Pulmonary orifice and valve.
Left anterior cusp
Right anterior cusp
Posterior cusp
Left ventricle
Nodule of valve
Left coronary artery
Nodule of valve
Auricle of left atrium
Left atrium
Accessory cusp
Anterior or aortic cusp of mitral valve
Posterior cusp of mitral valve
Left atrio-ventricular orifice and mitral valve
Interatrial septum

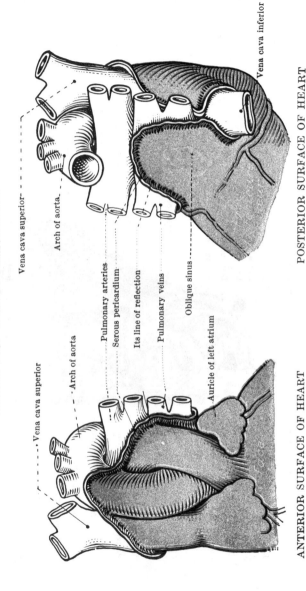

PLATE 193.—SEROUS PERICARDIUM

Vena cava superior

Arch of aorta

Pulmonary arteries

Serous pericardium

Its line of reflection

Pulmonary veins

Oblique sinus

Vena cava inferior

POSTERIOR SURFACE OF HEART

Vena cava superior

Arch of aorta

Auricle of left atrium

ANTERIOR SURFACE OF HEART

13

PLATE 194.—POSTERIOR WALL OF PERICARDIUM AFTER REMOVAL OF HEART

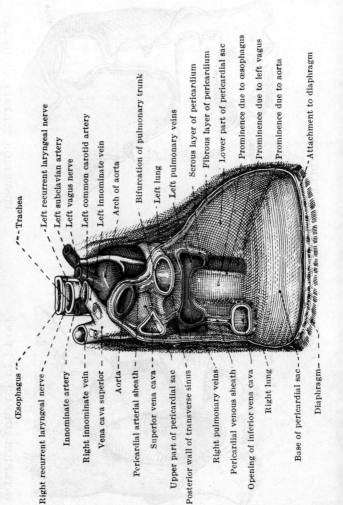

Œsophagus

Trachea

Left recurrent laryngeal nerve

Left subclavian artery

Left vagus nerve

Left common carotid artery

Left innominate vein

Arch of aorta

Bifurcation of pulmonary trunk

Left lung

Left pulmonary veins

Serous layer of pericardium

Fibrous layer of pericardium

Lower part of pericardial sac

Prominence due to œsophagus

Prominence due to left vagus

Prominence due to aorta

Attachment to diaphragm

Right recurrent laryngeal nerve

Innominate artery

Right innominate vein

Vena cava superior

Aorta

Pericardial arterial sheath

Superior vena cava

Upper part of pericardial sac

Posterior wall of transverse sinus

Right pulmonary veins

Pericardial venous sheath

Opening of inferior vena cava

Right lung

Base of pericardial sac

Diaphragm

PLATE 195.—DISSECTION OF ROOTS OF LUNGS AFTER REMOVAL OF POSTERIOR WALL OF PERICARDIUM

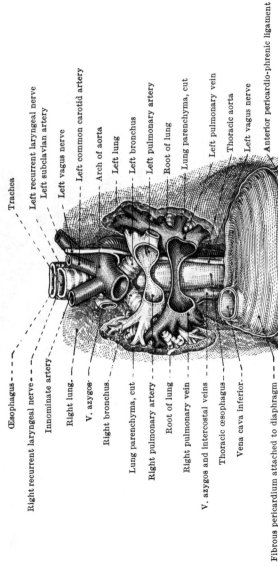

Œsophagus

Trachea

Right recurrent laryngeal nerve

Left recurrent laryngeal nerve

Innominate artery

Left subclavian artery

Right lung

Left vagus nerve

V. azygos

Left common carotid artery

Right bronchus

Arch of aorta

Left lung

Lung parenchyma, cut

Left bronchus

Right pulmonary artery

Left pulmonary artery

Root of lung

Root of lung

Right pulmonary vein

Lung parenchyma, cut

V. azygos and intercostal veins

Left pulmonary vein

Thoracic œsophagus

Thoracic aorta

Vena cava inferior

Left vagus nerve

Anterior pericardio-phrenic ligament

Fibrous pericardium attached to diaphragm

Diaphragm

PLATE 196.—CONTENTS OF MEDIASTINUM—SEEN FROM LEFT

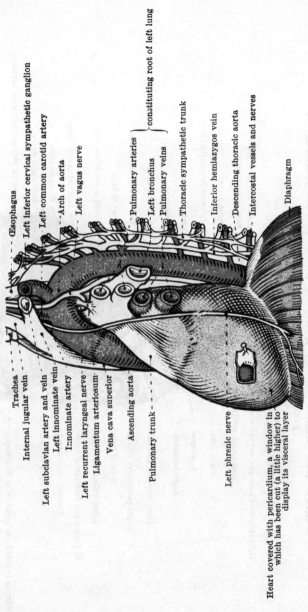

Trachea

Œsophagus

Internal jugular vein

Left inferior cervical sympathetic ganglion

Left subclavian artery and vein

Left common carotid artery

Left innominate vein

Arch of aorta

Innominate artery

Left vagus nerve

Left recurrent laryngeal nerve

Pulmonary arteries ⎫
Left bronchus ⎬ constituting root of left lung
Pulmonary veins ⎭

Ligamentum arteriosum

Vena cava superior

Thoracic sympathetic trunk

Ascending aorta

Inferior hemiazygos vein

Descending thoracic aorta

Intercostal vessels and nerves

Pulmonary trunk

Diaphragm

Left phrenic nerve

Heart covered with pericardium, a window in
which has been cut (a little higher) to
display its visceral layer

PLATE 197.—CONTENTS OF MEDIASTINUM—SEEN FROM RIGHT

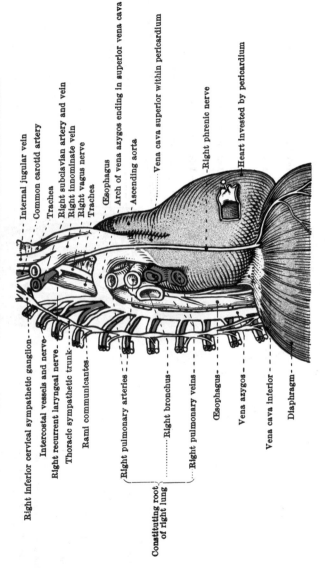

Right inferior cervical sympathetic ganglion

Internal jugular vein

Common carotid artery

Trachea

Intercostal vessels and nerve

Right subclavian artery and vein

Right recurrent laryngeal nerve

Right innominate vein

Thoracic sympathetic trunk

Right vagus nerve

Trachea

Rami communicantes

Œsophagus

Arch of vena azygos ending in superior vena cava

Ascending aorta

Vena cava superior within pericardium

Right phrenic nerve

Heart invested by pericardium

Right pulmonary arteries

Right bronchus

Constituting root of right lung

Right pulmonary veins

Œsophagus

Vena azygos

Vena cava inferior

Diaphragm

PLATE 198.—THYMUS AND ITS RELATIONS IN THE NEW-BORN

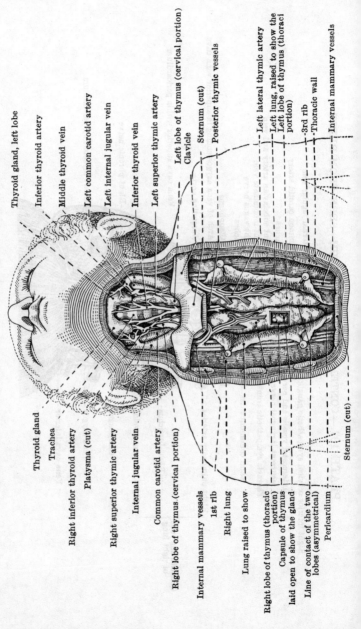

Thyroid gland, left lobe
Inferior thyroid artery
Middle thyroid vein
Left common carotid artery
Left internal jugular vein
Inferior thyroid vein
Left superior thymic artery
Left lobe of thymus (cervical portion)
Clavicle
Sternum (cut)
Posterior thymic vessels
Left lateral thymic artery
Left lung, raised to show the Left lobe of thymus (thoracic portion)
3rd rib
Thoracic wall
Internal mammary vessels

Thyroid gland
Trachea
Right inferior thyroid artery
Platysma (cut)
Right superior thymic artery
Internal jugular vein
Common carotid artery
Right lobe of thymus (cervical portion)
Internal mammary vessels
1st rib
Right lung
Lung raised to show
Right lobe of thymus (thoracic portion)
Capsule of thymus laid open to show the gland
Line of contact of the two lobes (asymmetrical)
Pericardium
Sternum (cut)

PLATE 199.—RELATIONS OF THYMUS
(HORIZONTAL SECTION AT THE LEVEL OF THE SECOND RIB)

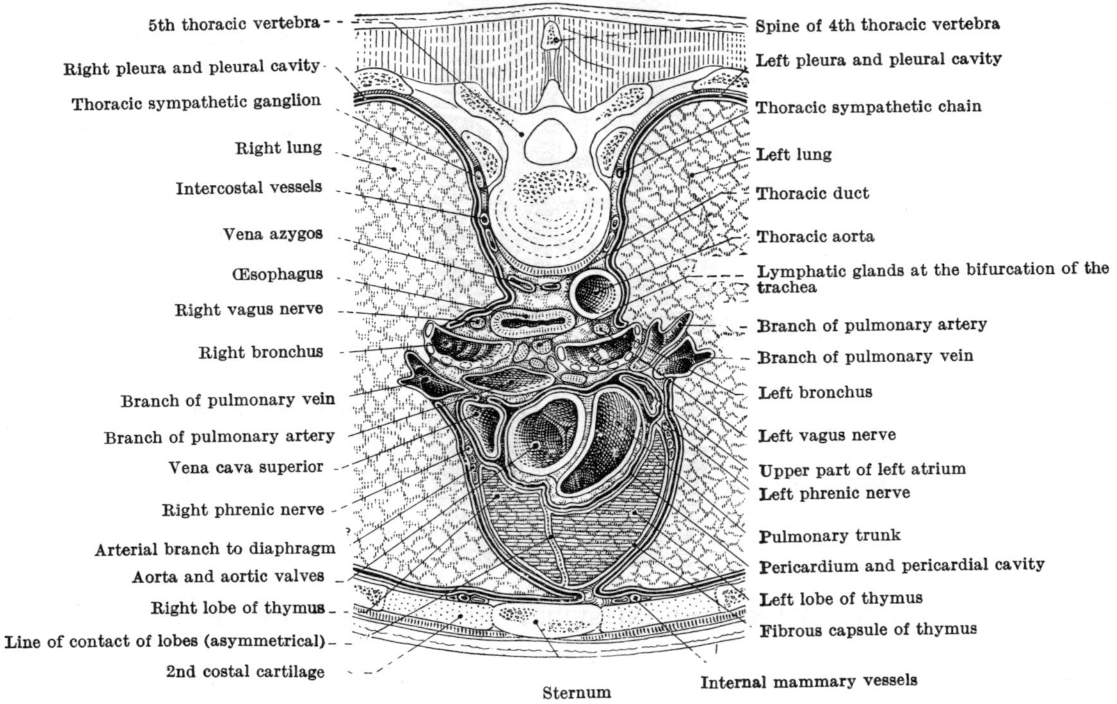

Labels (right side):
- Spine of 4th thoracic vertebra
- Left pleura and pleural cavity
- Thoracic sympathetic chain
- Left lung
- Thoracic duct
- Thoracic aorta
- Lymphatic glands at the bifurcation of the trachea
- Branch of pulmonary artery
- Branch of pulmonary vein
- Left bronchus
- Left vagus nerve
- Upper part of left atrium
- Left phrenic nerve
- Pulmonary trunk
- Pericardium and pericardial cavity
- Left lobe of thymus
- Fibrous capsule of thymus
- Internal mammary vessels

Labels (left side):
- 5th thoracic vertebra
- Right pleura and pleural cavity
- Thoracic sympathetic ganglion
- Right lung
- Intercostal vessels
- Vena azygos
- Œsophagus
- Right vagus nerve
- Right bronchus
- Branch of pulmonary vein
- Branch of pulmonary artery
- Vena cava superior
- Right phrenic nerve
- Arterial branch to diaphragm
- Aorta and aortic valves
- Right lobe of thymus
- Line of contact of lobes (asymmetrical)
- 2nd costal cartilage

Sternum

PLATE 200.—CONTENTS OF MEDIASTINUM—SEEN FROM BEHIND

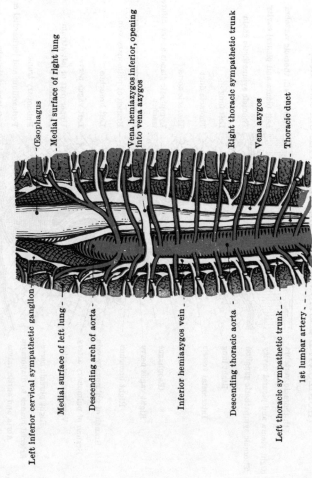

Left inferior cervical sympathetic ganglion

Medial surface of left lung

Descending arch of aorta

Inferior hemiazygos vein

Descending thoracic aorta

Left thoracic sympathetic trunk

1st lumbar artery

Œsophagus

Medial surface of right lung

Vena hemiazygos inferior, opening into vena azygos

Right thoracic sympathetic trunk

Vena azygos

Thoracic duct

PLATE 201.—CONTENTS OF MEDIASTINUM—SEEN FROM BEHIND [DEEPER DISSECTION]

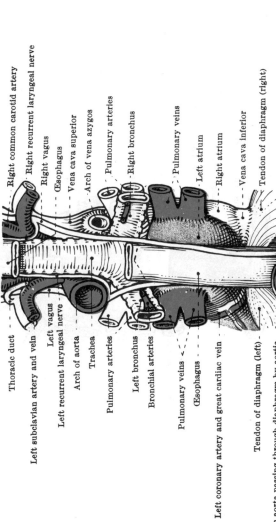

Thoracic duct

Left subclavian artery and vein

Left vagus

Left recurrent laryngeal nerve

Arch of aorta

Trachea

Pulmonary arteries

Left bronchus

Bronchial arteries

Pulmonary veins

Œsophagus

Left coronary artery and great cardiac vein

Tendon of diaphragm (left)

Thoracic aorta passing through diaphragm by aortic
opening with thoracic duct and vena azygos

Right common carotid artery

Right recurrent laryngeal nerve

Right vagus

Œsophagus

Vena cava superior

Arch of vena azygos

Pulmonary arteries

Right bronchus

Pulmonary veins

Left atrium

Right atrium

Vena cava inferior

Tendon of diaphragm (right)

Œsophageal opening (hiatus œsophageus), with right
and left vagi

PLATE 202.—CONTENTS OF MEDIASTINUM—SEEN FROM BEHIND [DEEPER DISSECTION]

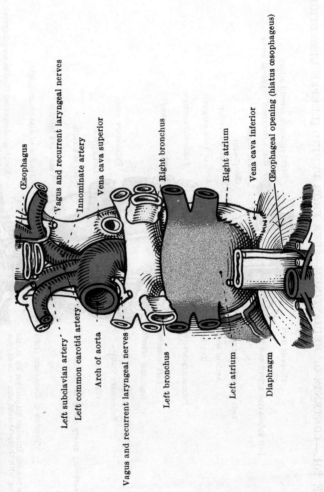

Œsophagus

Vagus and recurrent laryngeal nerves

Innominate artery

Vena cava superior

Right bronchus

Right atrium

Vena cava inferior

Œsophageal opening (hiatus œsophageus)

Left subclavian artery

Left common carotid artery

Arch of aorta

Vagus and recurrent laryngeal nerves

Left bronchus

Left atrium

Diaphragm

PLATE 203

ABDOMINAL AORTA AND ITS BRANCHES

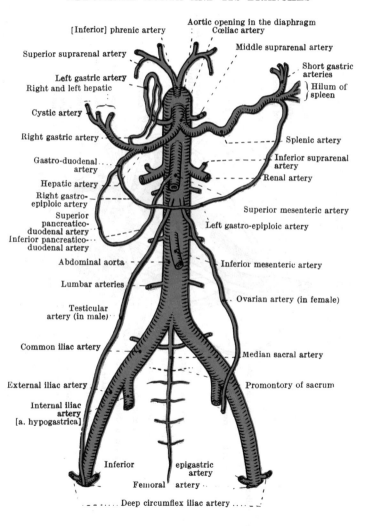

Aortic opening in the diaphragm
Cœliac artery

[Inferior] phrenic artery

Middle suprarenal artery

Superior suprarenal artery

Short gastric arteries

Left gastric artery
Right and left hepatic

Hilum of spleen

Cystic artery

Right gastric artery

Splenic artery

Gastro-duodenal artery

Inferior suprarenal artery

Hepatic artery

Renal artery

Right gastro-epiploic artery

Superior pancreatico-duodenal artery
Inferior pancreatico-duodenal artery

Superior mesenteric artery

Left gastro-epiploic artery

Abdominal aorta

Inferior mesenteric artery

Lumbar arteries

Ovarian artery (in female)

Testicular artery (in male)

Common iliac artery

Median sacral artery

External iliac artery

Promontory of sacrum

Internal iliac artery
[a. hypogastrica]

Inferior epigastric artery

Femoral artery

Deep circumflex iliac artery

PLATE 204.—VESSELS AND NERVES OF PELVIC CAVITY (MALE)

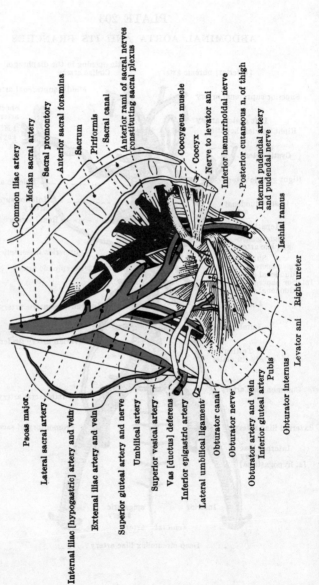

Common iliac artery
Median sacral artery
Sacral promontory
Anterior sacral foramina
Sacrum
Piriformis
Sacral canal
Anterior rami of sacral nerves constituting sacral plexus
Coccygeus muscle
Coccyx
Nerve to levator ani
Inferior hemorrhoidal nerve
Posterior cutaneous n. of thigh
Internal pudendal artery and pudendal nerve
Ischial ramus
Right ureter
Levator ani
Pubis
Obturator internus
Inferior gluteal artery
Obturator nerve
Obturator artery and vein
Lateral umbilical ligament
Inferior epigastric artery
Obturator canal
Vas [ductus] deferens
Superior vesical artery
Umbilical artery
Superior gluteal artery and nerve
External iliac artery and vein
Internal iliac [hypogastric] artery and vein
Lateral sacral artery
Psoas major

PLATE 205.—MALE PERINEUM

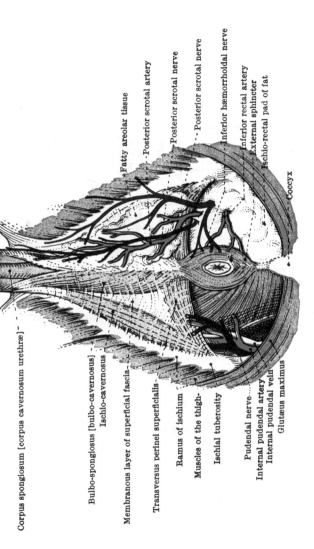

Corpus spongiosum [corpus cavernosum urethræ]
Bulbo-spongiosus [bulbo-cavernosus]
Ischio-cavernosus
Membranous layer of superficial fascia
Transversus perinei superficialis
Ramus of ischium
Muscles of the thigh
Ischial tuberosity
Pudendal nerve
Internal pudendal artery
Internal pudendal vein
Gluteus maximus

Fatty areolar tissue
Posterior scrotal artery
Posterior scrotal nerve
Posterior scrotal nerve
Inferior hæmorrhoidal nerve
Inferior rectal artery
External sphincter
Ischio-rectal pad of fat
Coccyx

PLATE 206.—RELATIONS OF ABDOMINAL VISCERA

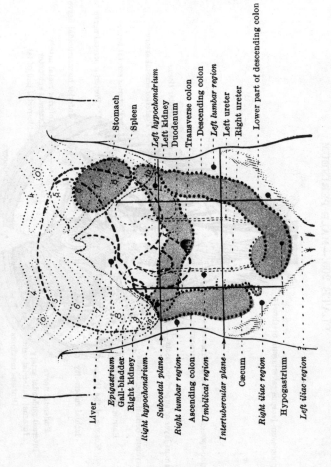

Liver
Epigastrium
Gall-bladder
Right kidney
Right hypochondrium
Subcostal plane
Right lumbar region
Ascending colon
Umbilical region
Intertubercular plane
Cæcum
Right iliac region
Hypogastrium
Left iliac region

Stomach
Spleen
Left hypochondrium
Left kidney
Duodenum
Transverse colon
Descending colon
Left lumbar region
Left ureter
Right ureter
Lower part of descending colon

PLATE 207.—RELATIONS OF ABDOMINAL VISCERA (*Continued*)

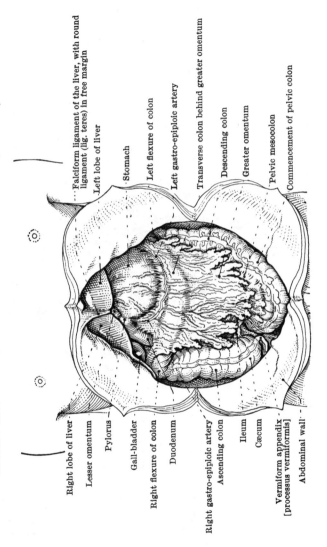

Falciform ligament of the liver, with round ligament (lig. teres) in free margin

Left lobe of liver

Stomach

Left flexure of colon

Left gastro-epiploic artery

Transverse colon behind greater omentum

Descending colon

Greater omentum

Pelvic mesocolon

Commencement of pelvic colon

Right lobe of liver

Lesser omentum

Pylorus

Gall-bladder

Right flexure of colon

Duodenum

Right gastro-epiploic artery

Ascending colon

Ileum

Cæcum

Vermiform appendix [processus vermiformis]

Abdominal wall

PLATE 208.—RELATIONS OF ABDOMINAL VISCERA (*Continued*)

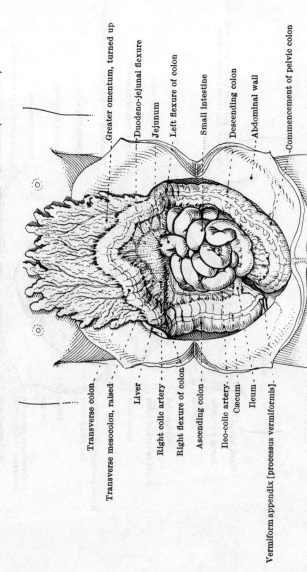

Greater omentum, turned up
Duodeno-jejunal flexure
Jejunum
Left flexure of colon
Small intestine
Descending colon
Abdominal wall
Commencement of pelvic colon

Transverse colon
Transverse mesocolon, raised
Liver
Right colic artery
Right flexure of colon
Ascending colon
Ileo-colic artery
Cæcum
Ileum
Vermiform appendix [processus vermiformis]

PLATE 209.—RELATIONS OF ABDOMINAL VISCERA (*Continued*)

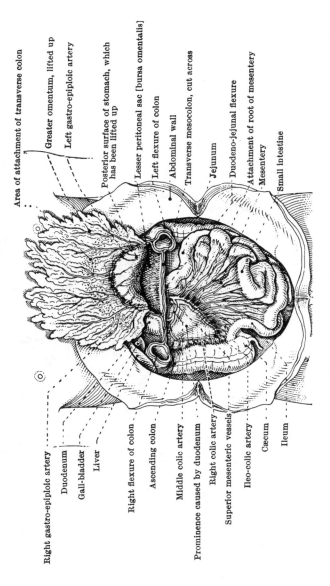

Area of attachment of transverse colon

Greater omentum, lifted up

Left gastro-epiploic artery

Posterior surface of stomach, which has been lifted up

Lesser peritoneal sac [bursa omentalis]

Left flexure of colon

Abdominal wall

Transverse mesocolon, cut across

Jejunum

Duodeno-jejunal flexure

Attachment of root of mesentery

Mesentery

Small intestine

Right gastro-epiploic artery

Duodenum

Gall-bladder

Liver

Right flexure of colon

Ascending colon

Middle colic artery

Prominence caused by duodenum

Right colic artery

Superior mesenteric vessels

Ileo-colic artery

Caecum

Ileum

14

PLATE 210.—RELATIONS OF ABDOMINAL VISCERA (*Continued*)

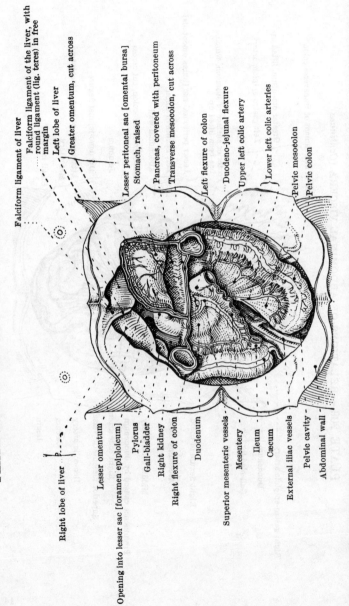

Falciform ligament of liver
Falciform ligament of the liver, with round ligament (lig. teres) in free margin
Left lobe of liver
Greater omentum, cut across
Lesser peritoneal sac [omental bursa]
Stomach, raised
Pancreas, covered with peritoneum
Transverse mesocolon, cut across
Left flexure of colon
Duodeno-jejunal flexure
Upper left colic artery
Lower left colic artery
Pelvic mesocolon
Pelvic colon

Right lobe of liver
Lesser omentum
Opening into lesser sac [foramen epiploicum]
Pylorus
Gall-bladder
Right kidney
Right flexure of colon
Duodenum
Superior mesenteric vessels
Mesentery
Ileum
Caecum
External iliac vessels
Pelvic cavity
Abdominal wall

PLATE 211.—RELATIONS OF ABDOMINAL VISCERA (Continued)

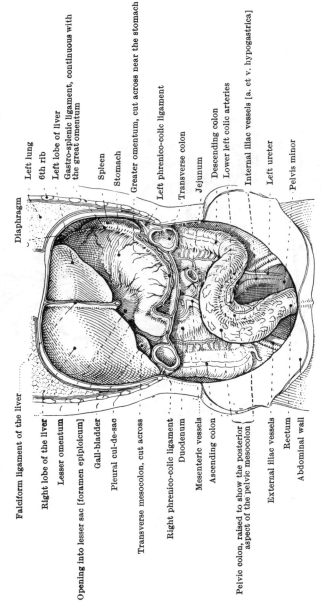

Falciform ligament of the liver

Right lobe of the liver

Lesser omentum

Opening into lesser sac [foramen epiploicum]

Gall-bladder

Pleural cul-de-sac

Transverse mesocolon, cut across

Right phrenico-colic ligament

Duodenum

Mesenteric vessels

Ascending colon

Pelvic colon, raised to show the posterior aspect of the pelvic mesocolon

External iliac vessels

Rectum

Abdominal wall

Diaphragm

Left lung

6th rib

Left lobe of liver

Gastro-splenic ligament, continuous with the great omentum

Spleen

Stomach

Greater omentum, cut across near the stomach

Left phrenico-colic ligament

Transverse colon

Jejunum

Descending colon

Lower left colic arteries

Internal iliac vessels [a. et v. hypogastrica]

Left ureter

Pelvis minor

PLATE 212.—RELATIONS OF ABDOMINAL VISCERA (*Continued*)

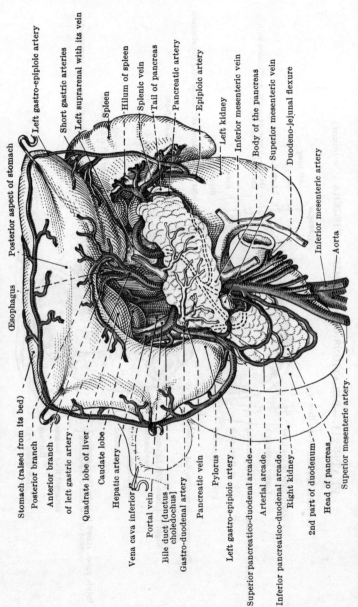

Œsophagus

Posterior aspect of stomach

Left gastro-epiploïc artery

Short gastric arteries

Left suprarenal with its vein

Spleen

Hilum of spleen

Splenic vein

Tail of pancreas

Pancreatic artery

Epiploïc artery

Left kidney

Inferior mesenteric vein

Body of the pancreas

Superior mesenteric vein

Duodeno-jejunal flexure

Inferior mesenteric artery

Aorta

Stomach (raised from its bed)

Posterior branch

Anterior branch

of left gastric artery

Quadrate lobe of liver

Caudate lobe

Hepatic artery

Vena cava inferior

Portal vein

Bile duct [ductus choledochus]

Gastro-duodenal artery

Pancreatic vein

Pylorus

Left gastro-epiploic artery

Superior pancreatico-duodenal arcade

Arterial arcade

Inferior pancreatico-duodenal arcade

Right kidney

2nd part of duodenum

Head of pancreas

Superior mesenteric artery

PLATE 213.—RELATIONS OF ABDOMINAL VISCERA (Continued)

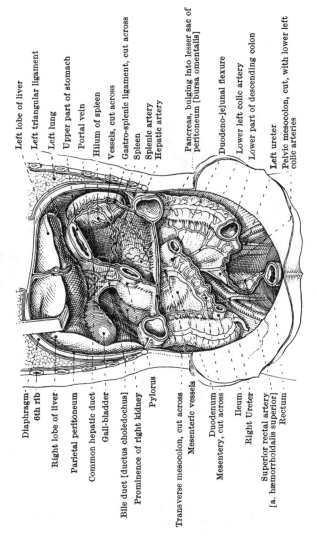

Left lobe of liver
Left triangular ligament
Left lung
Upper part of stomach
Portal vein
Hilum of spleen
Vessels, cut across
Gastro-splenic ligament, cut across
Spleen
Splenic artery
Hepatic artery

Pancreas, bulging into lesser sac of peritoneum [bursa omentalis]
Duodeno-jejunal flexure
Lower left colic artery
Lower part of descending colon

Left ureter
Pelvic mesocolon, cut, with lower left colic arteries

Diaphragm
6th rib

Right lobe of liver

Parietal peritoneum

Common hepatic duct
Gall-bladder

Bile duct [ductus choledochus]
Prominence of right kidney

Pylorus

Transverse mesocolon, cut across
Mesenteric vessels

Duodenum
Mesentery, cut across

Ileum
Right Ureter

Superior rectal artery
[a. hæmorrhoidalis superior]
Rectum

PLATE 214.—RELATIONS OF ABDOMINAL VISCERA (*Continued*)

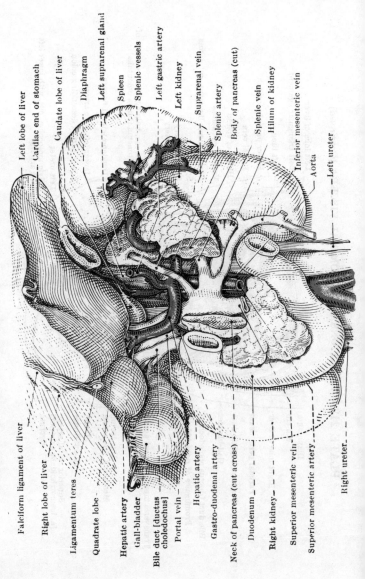

Left lobe of liver

Cardiac end of stomach

Caudate lobe of liver

Diaphragm

Left suprarenal gland

Spleen

Splenic vessels

Left gastric artery

Left kidney

Suprarenal vein

Splenic artery

Body of pancreas (cut)

Splenic vein

Hilum of kidney

Inferior mesenteric vein

Aorta

Left ureter

Faleiform ligament of liver

Right lobe of liver

Ligamentum teres

Quadrate lobe

Hepatic artery

Gall-bladder

Bile duct [ductus choledochus]

Portal vein

Hepatic artery

Gastro-duodenal artery

Neck of pancreas (cut across)

Duodenum

Right kidney

Superior mesenteric vein

Superior mesenteric artery

Right ureter

PLATE 215.—RELATIONS OF ABDOMINAL VISCERA (*Continued*)

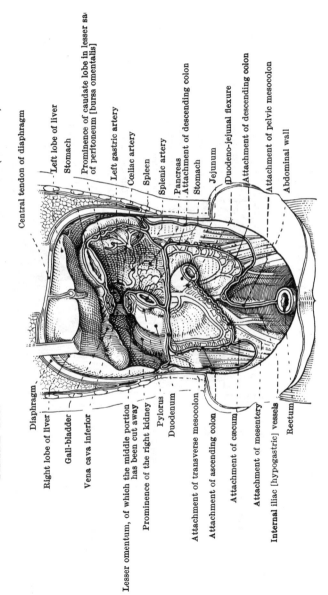

Central tendon of diaphragm

Left lobe of liver

Stomach

Prominence of caudate lobe in lesser sac of peritoneum [bursa omentalis]

Left gastric artery

Celiac artery

Spleen

Splenic artery

Pancreas

Attachment of descending colon

Stomach

Jejunum

Duodeno-jejunal flexure

Attachment of descending colon

Attachment of pelvic mesocolon

Abdominal wall

Diaphragm

Right lobe of liver

Gall-bladder

Vena cava inferior

Lesser omentum, of which the middle portion has been cut away

Prominence of the right kidney

Pylorus

Duodenum

Attachment of transverse mesocolon

Attachment of ascending colon

Attachment of cæcum

Attachment of mesentery

Internal iliac [hypogastric] vessels

Rectum

PLATE 216.—RELATIONS OF ABDOMINAL VISCERA (Continued)

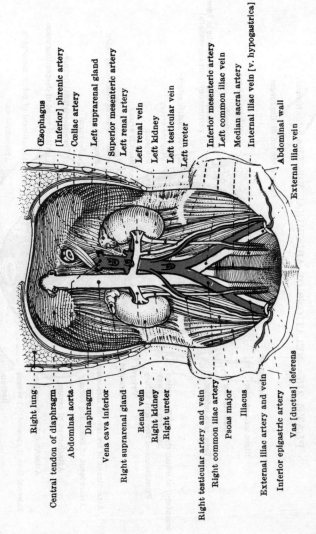

Right lung

Central tendon of diaphragm

Abdominal aorta

Diaphragm

Vena cava inferior

Right suprarenal gland

Renal vein

Right kidney

Right ureter

Right testicular artery and vein

Right common iliac artery

Psoas major

Iliacus

External iliac artery and vein

Inferior epigastric artery

Vas [ductus] deferens

Œsophagus

[Inferior] phrenic artery

Cœliac artery

Left suprarenal gland

Superior mesenteric artery

Left renal artery

Left renal vein

Left kidney

Left testicular vein

Left ureter

Inferior mesenteric artery

Left common iliac vein

Median sacral artery

Internal iliac vein [v. hypogastrica]

Abdominal wall

External iliac vein

PLATE 217.—CŒLIAC PLEXUS

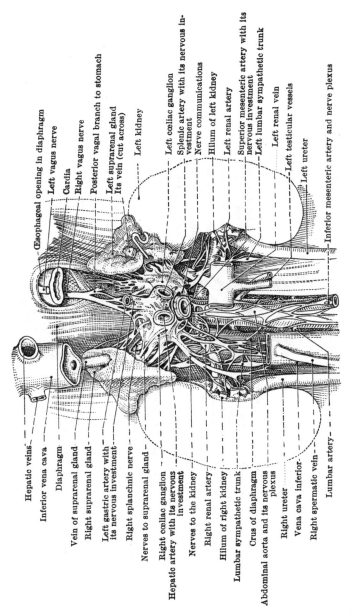

Œsophageal opening in diaphragm
Left vagus nerve
Cardia
Right vagus nerve
Posterior vagal branch to stomach
Left suprarenal gland
Its vein (cut across)
Left kidney

Left cœliac ganglion
Splenic artery with its nervous in-
vestment
Nerve communications
Hilum of left kidney
Left renal artery
Superior mesenteric artery with its
nervous investment
Left lumbar sympathetic trunk
Left renal vein
Left testicular vessels
Left ureter
Inferior mesenteric artery and nerve plexus

Hepatic veins
Inferior vena cava
Diaphragm
Vein of suprarenal gland
Right suprarenal gland
Left gastric artery with
its nervous investment
Right splanchnic nerve
Nerves to suprarenal gland
Right cœliac ganglion
Hepatic artery with its nervous
investment
Nerves to the kidney
Right renal artery
Hilum of right kidney
Lumbar sympathetic trunk
Crus of diaphragm
Abdominal aorta and its nervous
plexus
Right ureter
Vena cava inferior
Right spermatic vein
Lumbar artery

PLATE 218.—PERITONEUM—MEDIAN SECTION OF MALE BODY

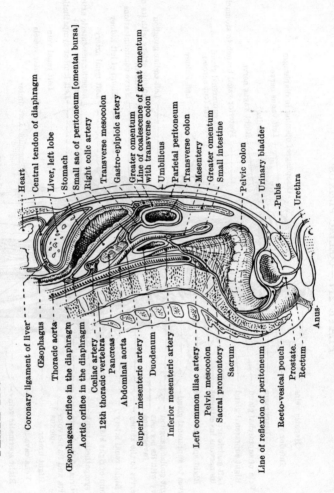

Coronary ligament of liver
Œsophagus
Thoracic aorta
Œsophageal orifice in the diaphragm
Aortic orifice in the diaphragm
Cœliac artery
12th thoracic vertebra
Pancreas
Abdominal aorta
Superior mesenteric artery
Duodenum
Inferior mesenteric artery
Left common iliac artery
Pelvic mesocolon
Sacral promontory
Sacrum
Line of reflexion of peritoneum
Recto-vesical pouch
Prostate
Rectum

Heart
Central tendon of diaphragm
Liver, left lobe
Stomach
Small sac of peritoneum [omental bursa]
Right colic artery
Transverse mesocolon
Gastro-epiploic artery
Greater omentum
Line of coalescence of great omentum with transverse colon
Umbilicus
Parietal peritoneum
Transverse colon
Mesentery
Greater omentum
Small intestine
Pelvic colon
Urinary bladder
Pubis
Urethra
Anus

PLATE 219.—SPLEEN

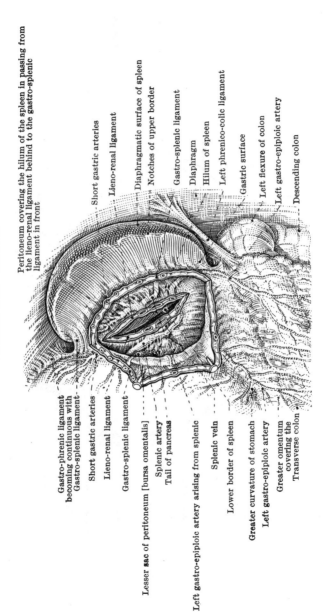

Peritoneum covering the hilum of the spleen in passing from the lieno-renal ligament behind to the gastro-splenic ligament in front

Short gastric arteries

Lieno-renal ligament

Diaphragmatic surface of spleen

Notches of upper border

Gastro-splenic ligament

Diaphragm

Hilum of spleen

Left phrenico-colic ligament

Gastric surface

Left flexure of colon

Left gastro-epiploic artery

Descending colon

Gastro-phrenic ligament becoming continuous with Gastro-splenic ligament

Short gastric arteries

Lieno-renal ligament

Gastro-splenic ligament

Lesser sac of peritoneum [bursa omentalis]

Splenic artery

Tail of pancreas

Left gastro-epiploic artery arising from splenic

Splenic vein

Lower border of spleen

Greater curvature of stomach

Left gastro-epiploic artery

Greater omentum covering the Transverse colon

PLATE 220.—LIVER—SEEN FROM BELOW

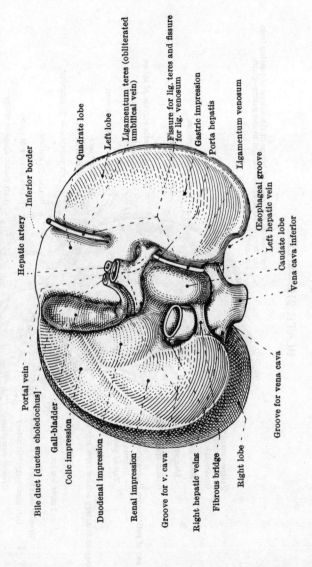

Hepatic artery
Inferior border
Portal vein
Bile duct [ductus choledochus]
Gall-bladder
Colic impression
Duodenal impression
Renal impression
Groove for v. cava
Right hepatic veins
Fibrous bridge
Right lobe
Groove for vena cava
Quadrate lobe
Left lobe
Ligamentum teres (obliterated umbilical vein)
Fissure for lig. teres and fissure for lig. venosum
Gastric impression
Porta hepatis
Ligamentum venosum
Œsophageal groove
Left hepatic vein
Caudate lobe
Vena cava inferior

PLATE 221.—LIVER (*Continued*)

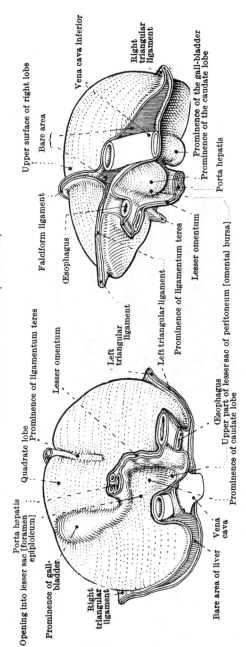

Porta hepatis [foramen epiploicum]

Opening into lesser sac

Prominence of gall-bladder

Right triangular ligament

Bare area of liver

Vena cava

Prominence of caudate lobe

Quadrate lobe

Prominence of ligamentum teres

Lesser omentum

Left triangular ligament

Œsophagus

Upper part of lesser sac of peritoneum [omental bursa]

INFERIOR ASPECT

Upper surface of right lobe

Bare area

Vena cava inferior

Falciform ligament

Œsophagus

Prominence of ligamentum teres

Lesser omentum

Right triangular ligament

Prominence of the gall-bladder

Prominence of the caudate lobe

Porta hepatis

POSTERIOR ASPECT

PLATE 222.—PANCREAS

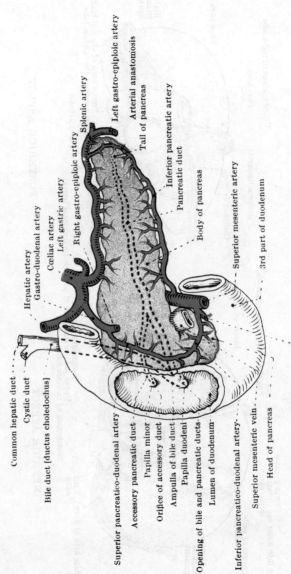

Common hepatic duct
Cystic duct
Bile duct [ductus choledochus]

Superior pancreatico-duodenal artery
Accessory pancreatic duct
Papilla minor
Orifice of accessory duct
Ampulla of bile duct
Papilla duodeni
Opening of bile and pancreatic ducts
Lumen of duodenum

Inferior pancreatico-duodenal artery
Superior mesenteric vein
Head of pancreas

Posterior pancreatic artery

Hepatic artery
Gastro-duodenal artery
Cœliac artery
Left gastric artery
Right gastro-epiploic artery
Splenic artery

Left gastro-epiploic artery
Arterial anastomosis
Tail of pancreas

Inferior pancreatic artery
Pancreatic duct

Body of pancreas

Superior mesenteric artery

3rd part of duodenum

PLATE 223.—DUODENO-JEJUNAL FLEXURE

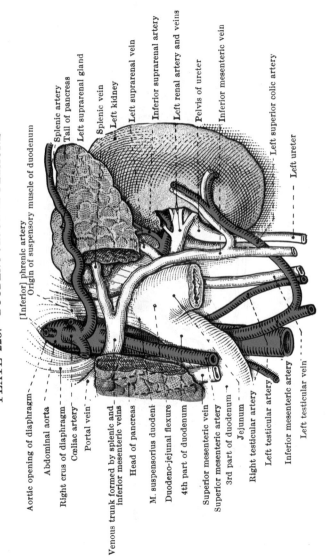

Aortic opening of diaphragm
Abdominal aorta
Right crus of diaphragm
Cœliac artery
Portal vein
Venous trunk formed by splenic and inferior mesenteric veins
Head of pancreas
M. suspensorius duodeni
Duodeno-jejunal flexure
4th part of duodenum
Superior mesenteric vein
Superior mesenteric artery
3rd part of duodenum
Jejunum
Right testicular artery
Left testicular artery
Inferior mesenteric artery
Left testicular vein

[Inferior] phrenic artery
Origin of suspensory muscle of duodenum
Splenic artery
Tail of pancreas
Left suprarenal gland
Splenic vein
Left kidney
Left suprarenal vein

Inferior suprarenal artery
Left renal artery and veins
Pelvis of ureter
Inferior mesenteric vein

Left superior colic artery
Left ureter

PLATE 224.—HORIZONTAL SECTION THROUGH TRUNK

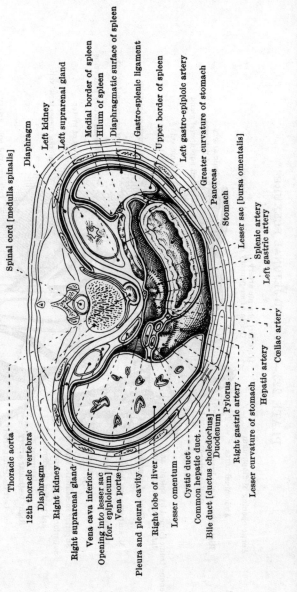

Spinal cord [medulla spinalis]

Diaphragm

Left kidney

Left suprarenal gland

Medial border of spleen

Hilum of spleen

Diaphragmatic surface of spleen

Gastro-splenic ligament

Upper border of spleen

Left gastro-epiploic artery

Greater curvature of stomach

Pancreas

Stomach

Lesser sac [bursa omentalis]

Splenic artery

Left gastric artery

Coeliac artery

Hepatic artery

Right gastric artery

Lesser curvature of stomach

Duodenum

Bile duct [ductus choledochus]

Common hepatic duct

Cystic duct

Lesser omentum

Right lobe of liver

Pleura and pleural cavity

Opening into lesser sac [for. epiploicum]

Vena portae

Vena cava inferior

Right suprarenal gland

Right kidney

Diaphragm

12th thoracic vertebra

Thoracic aorta

Pylorus

PLATE 225.—LESSER SAC OF PERITONEUM [BURSA OMENTALIS] IN HORIZONTAL SECTION

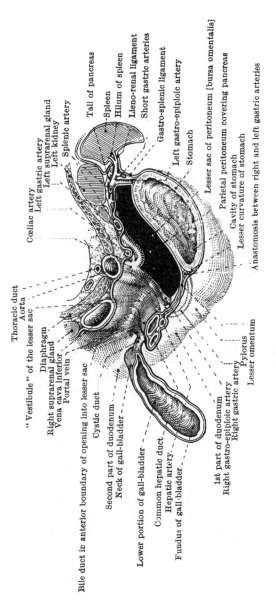

Thoracic duct
Aorta
Diaphragm
"Vestibule" of the lesser sac
Right suprarenal gland
Vena cava inferior
Portal vein

Celiac artery
Left gastric artery
Left suprarenal gland
Left kidney
Splenic artery

Tail of pancreas
Spleen
Hilum of spleen
Lieno-renal ligament
Short gastric arteries
Gastro-splenic ligament
Left gastro-epiploic artery
Stomach
Lesser sac of peritoneum [bursa omentalis]
Parietal peritoneum covering pancreas
Cavity of stomach
Lesser curvature of stomach
Anastomosis between right and left gastric arteries

Bile duct in anterior boundary of opening into lesser sac
Cystic duct
Second part of duodenum
Neck of gall-bladder
Lower portion of gall-bladder
Common hepatic duct
Hepatic artery
Fundus of gall-bladder
1st part of duodenum
Right gastro-epiploic artery
Right gastric artery
Pylorus
Lesser omentum

15

PLATE 226.—LESSER OMENTUM

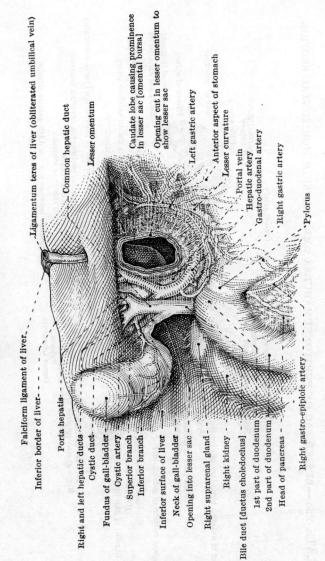

Faleiform ligament of liver

Ligamentum teres of liver (obliterated umbilical vein)

Inferior border of liver

Common hepatic duct

Lesser omentum

Porta hepatis

Caudate lobe causing prominence in lesser sac [omental bursa]

Opening cut in lesser omentum to show lesser sac

Right and left hepatic ducts

Cystic duct

Fundus of gall-bladder

Cystic artery

Superior branch

Inferior branch

Left gastric artery

Anterior aspect of stomach

Lesser curvature

Portal vein

Hepatic artery

Gastro-duodenal artery

Right gastric artery

Inferior surface of liver

Neck of gall-bladder

Opening into lesser sac

Right suprarenal gland

Right kidney

Bile duct [ductus choledochus]

1st part of duodenum

2nd part of duodenum

Head of pancreas

Right gastro-epiploic artery

Pylorus

PLATE 227.—DUODENUM

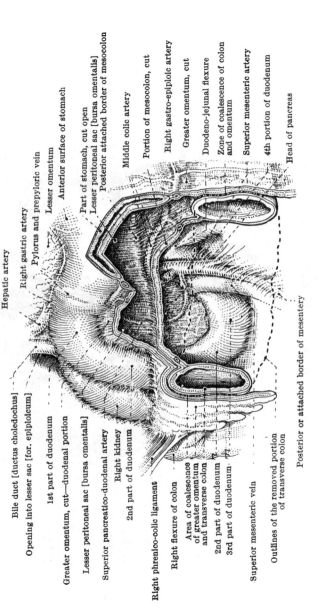

Bile duct [ductus choledochus]
Opening into lesser sac [for. epiploeum]
1st part of duodenum
Greater omentum, cut—duodenal portion
Lesser peritoneal sac [bursa omentalis]
Superior pancreatico-duodenal artery
Right kidney
2nd part of duodenum

Right phrenico-colic ligament
Right flexure of colon
Area of coalescence of greater omentum and transverse colon
2nd part of duodenum
3rd part of duodenum

Superior mesenteric vein

Outlines of the removed portion of transverse colon

Posterior or attached border of mesentery

Hepatic artery
Right gastric artery
Pylorus and prepyloric vein
Lesser omentum
Anterior surface of stomach
Part of stomach, cut open
Lesser peritoneal sac [bursa omentalis]
Posterior attached border of mesocolon

Middle colic artery
Portion of mesocolon, cut
Right gastro-epiploic artery
Greater omentum, cut
Duodeno-jejunal flexure
Zone of coalescence of colon and omentum
Superior mesenteric artery
4th portion of duodenum
Head of pancreas

PLATE 228.—KIDNEYS AND SUPRARENAL GLANDS

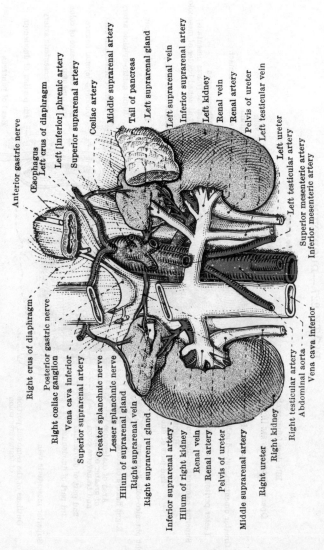

Right crus of diaphragm

Anterior gastric nerve

Œsophagus
Left crus of diaphragm
Left [inferior] phrenic artery
Superior suprarenal artery
Cœliac artery
Middle suprarenal artery
Left suprarenal gland
Tail of pancreas
Left suprarenal gland
Left suprarenal vein
Inferior suprarenal artery
Left kidney
Renal vein
Renal artery
Pelvis of ureter
Left testicular vein
Left ureter
Left testicular artery
Superior mesenteric artery
Inferior mesenteric artery

Posterior gastric nerve
Right cœliac ganglion
Vena cava inferior
Superior suprarenal artery
Greater splanchnic nerve
Lesser splanchnic nerve
Hilum of suprarenal gland
Right suprarenal vein
Right suprarenal gland

Inferior suprarenal artery
Hilum of right kidney
Renal vein
Renal artery
Pelvis of ureter

Middle suprarenal artery

Right ureter
Right kidney

Right testicular artery
Abdominal aorta
Vena cava inferior

PLATE 229.—VERTICAL SECTION OF RIGHT KIDNEY

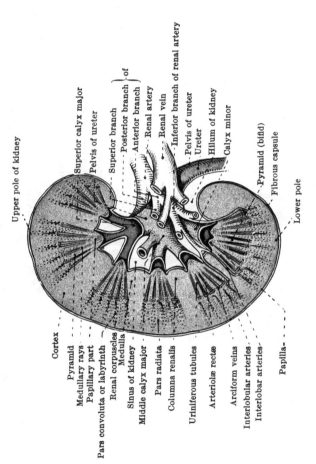

Upper pole of kidney

Superior calyx major
Pelvis of ureter
Superior branch
Posterior branch ⎤ of
Anterior branch ⎦
Renal artery
Renal vein
Inferior branch of renal artery
Pelvis of ureter
Ureter
Hilum of kidney
Calyx minor

Pyramid (bifid)
Fibrous capsule

Lower pole

Cortex
Pyramid
Medullary rays
Papillary part
Pars convoluta or labyrinth
Renal corpuscles
Medulla
Sinus of kidney
Middle calyx major
Pars radiata
Columna renalis
Uriniferous tubules
Arteriolæ rectæ
Arciform veins
Interlobular arteries
Interlobar arteries
Papilla

PLATE 230.—LUMBAR PLEXUS

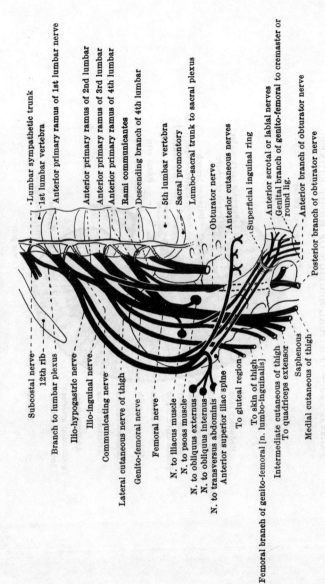

Lumbar sympathetic trunk
1st lumbar vertebra
Anterior primary ramus of 1st lumbar nerve
Anterior primary ramus of 2nd lumbar
Anterior primary ramus of 3rd lumbar
Anterior primary ramus of 4th lumbar
Rami communicantes
Descending branch of 4th lumbar
5th lumbar vertebra
Sacral promontory
Lumbo-sacral trunk to sacral plexus
Obturator nerve
Anterior cutaneous nerves
Superficial inguinal ring
Anterior scrotal or labial nerves
Genital branch of genito-femoral to cremaster or round lig.
Anterior branch of obturator nerve
Posterior branch of obturator nerve

Subcostal nerve
12th rib
Branch to lumbar plexus
Ilio-hypogastric nerve
Ilio-inguinal nerve
Communicating nerve
Lateral cutaneous nerve of thigh
Genito-femoral nerve
Femoral nerve
N. to iliacus muscle
N. to psoas muscle
N. to obliquus externus
N. to obliquus internus
N. to transversus abdominis
Anterior superior iliac spine
To gluteal region
To skin of thigh
Femoral branch of genito-femoral [n. lumbo-inguinalis]
Intermediate cutaneous of thigh
To quadriceps extensor
Saphenous
Medial cutaneous of thigh

PLATE 231.—SACRAL PLEXUS

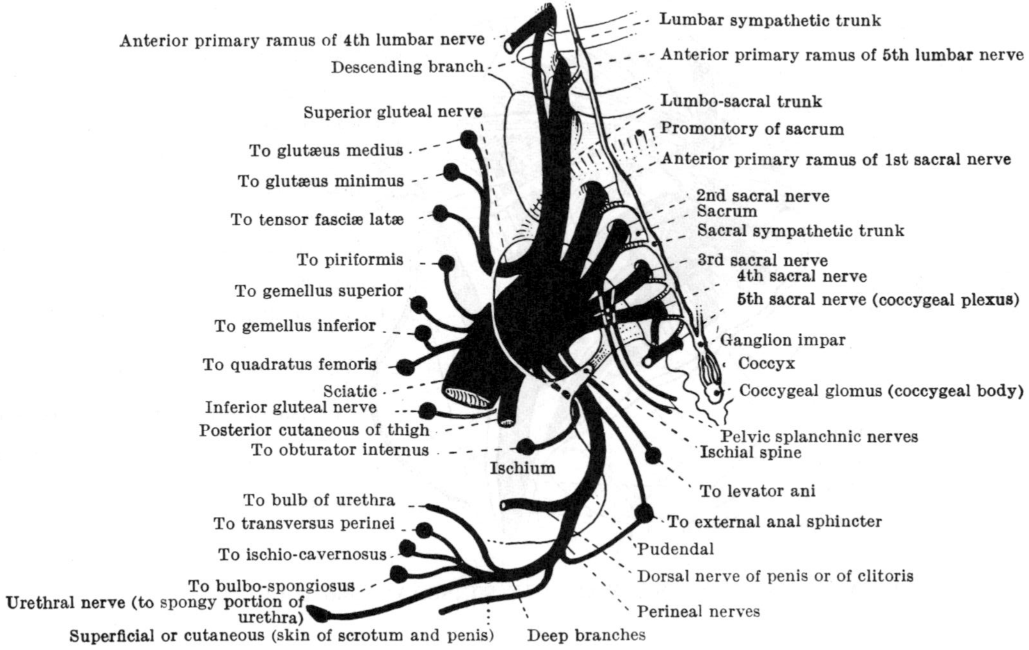

Lumbar sympathetic trunk
Anterior primary ramus of 5th lumbar nerve
Lumbo-sacral trunk
Promontory of sacrum
Anterior primary ramus of 1st sacral nerve
2nd sacral nerve
Sacrum
Sacral sympathetic trunk
3rd sacral nerve
4th sacral nerve
5th sacral nerve (coccygeal plexus)
Ganglion impar
Coccyx
Coccygeal glomus (coccygeal body)
Ischial spine
Pelvic splanchnic nerves
To levator ani
To external anal sphincter
Pudendal
Dorsal nerve of penis or of clitoris
Perineal nerves

Anterior primary ramus of 4th lumbar nerve
Descending branch
Superior gluteal nerve
To gluteus medius
To gluteus minimus
To tensor fasciae latae
To piriformis
To gemellus superior
To quadratus femoris
Sciatic
Inferior gluteal nerve
Posterior cutaneous of thigh
To obturator internus

Ischium

Deep branches

To bulb of urethra
To transversus perinei
To ischio-cavernosus

Urethral nerve (to spongy portion of urethra)
To bulbo-spongiosus
Superficial or cutaneous (skin of scrotum and penis)

PLATE 232.—VESSELS AND NERVES OF PELVIC CAVITY (MALE)

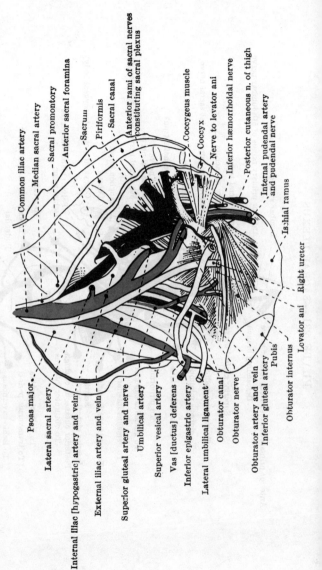

Common iliac artery
Median sacral artery
Sacral promontory
Anterior sacral foramina
Sacrum
Piriformis
Sacral canal
Anterior rami of sacral nerves constituting sacral plexus
Coccygeus muscle
Coccyx
Nerve to levator ani
Inferior hæmorrhoidal nerve
Posterior cutaneous n. of thigh
Internal pudendal artery and pudendal nerve
Ischial ramus
Right ureter
Levator ani
Pubis
Obturator internus
Inferior gluteal artery
Obturator artery and vein
Obturator nerve
Obturator canal
Lateral umbilical ligament
Inferior epigastric artery
Vas [ductus] deferens
Superior vesical artery
Umbilical artery
Superior gluteal artery and nerve
External iliac artery and vein
Internal iliac [hypogastric] artery and vein
Lateral sacral artery and vein
Psoas major

PLATE 233.—ARTERIES OF PELVIC CAVITY (MALE)

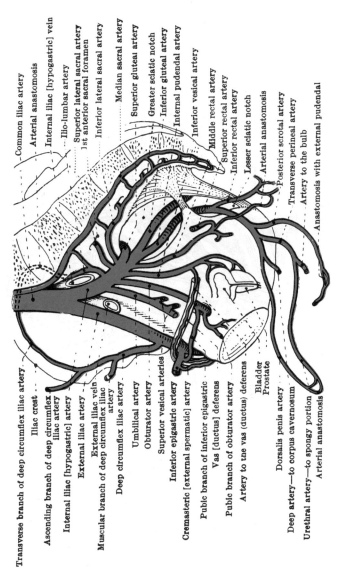

Transverse branch of deep circumflex iliac artery

Iliac crest

Ascending branch of deep circumflex iliac artery

Internal iliac [hypogastric] artery

External iliac artery

External iliac vein

Muscular branch of deep circumflex iliac artery

Deep circumflex iliac artery

Umbilical artery

Obturator artery

Superior vesical arteries

Inferior epigastric artery

Cremasteric [external spermatic] artery

Pubic branch of inferior epigastric

Vas [ductus] deferens

Pubic branch of obturator artery

Artery to the vas (ductus) deferens

Bladder

Prostate

Dorsalis penis artery

Deep artery—to corpus cavernosum

Urethral artery—to spongy portion

Arterial anastomosis

Common iliac artery

Arterial anastomosis

Internal iliac [hypogastric] vein

Ilio-lumbar artery

Superior lateral sacral artery

1st anterior sacral foramen

Inferior lateral sacral artery

Median sacral artery

Superior gluteal artery

Greater sciatic notch

Inferior gluteal artery

Internal pudendal artery

Inferior vesical artery

Middle rectal artery

Superior rectal artery

Inferior rectal artery

Lesser sciatic notch

Arterial anastomosis

Posterior scrotal artery

Transverse perineal artery

Artery to the bulb

Anastomosis with external pudendal

PLATE 234.—PERITONEUM—MEDIAN SECTION OF MALE BODY

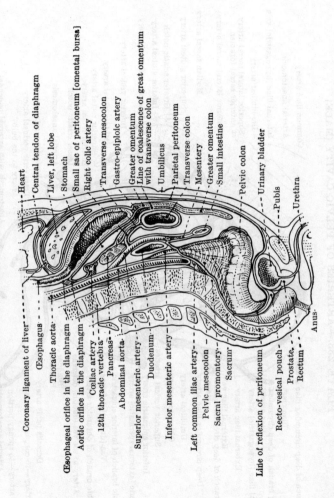

Heart
Central tendon of diaphragm
Liver, left lobe
Stomach
Small sac of peritoneum [omental bursa]
Right colic artery
Transverse mesocolon
Gastro-epiploic artery
Greater omentum
Line of coalescence of great omentum with transverse colon
Umbilicus
Parietal peritoneum
Transverse colon
Mesentery
Greater omentum
Small intestine
Pelvic colon
Urinary bladder
Pubis
Urethra
Anus

Coronary ligament of liver
Œsophagus
Thoracic aorta
Œsophageal orifice in the diaphragm
Aortic orifice in the diaphragm
Cœliac artery
12th thoracic vertebra
Pancreas
Abdominal aorta
Superior mesenteric artery
Duodenum
Inferior mesenteric artery
Left common iliac artery
Pelvic mesocolon
Sacral promontory
Sacrum
Line of reflexion of peritoneum
Recto-vesical pouch
Prostate
Rectum

PLATE 235.—PORTAL VEIN AND ITS TRIBUTARIES

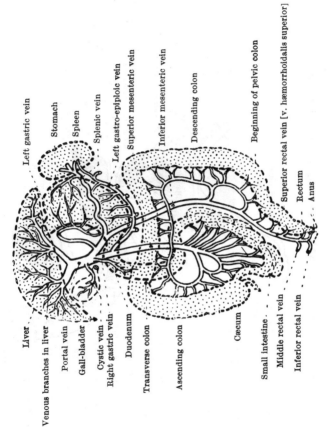

Liver
Venous branches in liver
Portal vein
Gall-bladder
Cystic vein
Right gastric vein
Duodenum
Transverse colon
Ascending colon
Caecum
Small intestine
Middle rectal vein
Inferior rectal vein

Left gastric vein
Stomach
Spleen
Splenic vein
Left gastro-epiploic vein
Superior mesenteric vein
Inferior mesenteric vein
Descending colon
Beginning of pelvic colon
Superior rectal vein [v. hemorrhoidalis superior]
Rectum
Anus

PLATE 236.—DIAGRAM OF MALE GENITAL ORGANS

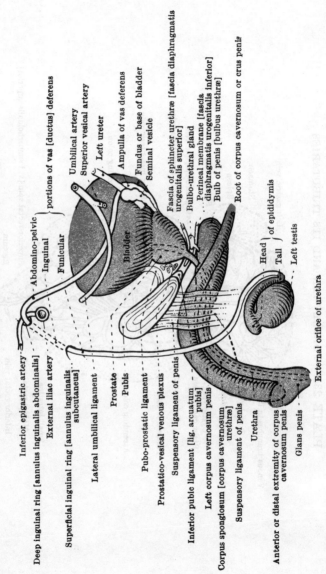

Inferior epigastric artery

Deep inguinal ring [annulus inguinalis abdominalis]

External iliac artery

Superficial inguinal ring [annulus inguinalis subcutaneus]

Lateral umbilical ligament

Prostate

Pubis

Pubo-prostatic ligament

Prostatico-vesical venous plexus

Suspensory ligament of penis

Inferior pubic ligament [lig. arcuatum pubis]

Left corpus cavernosum penis

Corpus spongiosum [corpus cavernosum urethræ]

Suspensory ligament of penis

Urethra

Anterior or distal extremity of corpus cavernosum penis

Glans penis

External orifice of urethra

Abdomino-pelvic
Inguinal
Funicular

portions of vas [ductus] deferens

Umbilical artery

Superior vesical artery

Left ureter

Ampulla of vas deferens

Fundus or base of bladder

Seminal vesicle

Bladder

Fascia of sphincter urethræ [fascia diaphragmatis urogenitalis superior]

Bulbo-urethral gland

Perineal membrane [fascia diaphragmatis urogenitalis inferior]

Bulb of penis [bulbus urethræ]

Root of corpus cavernosum or crus penis

Head
Tail

of epididymis

Left testis

PLATE 237.—MALE URETHRA, LAID OPEN

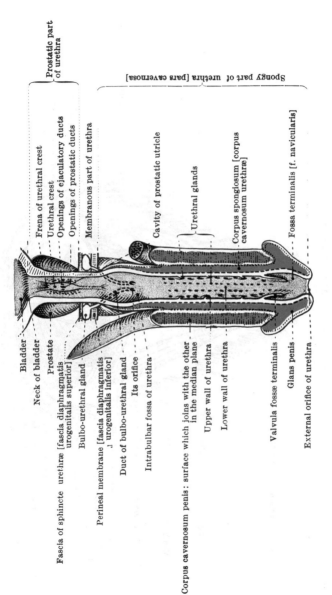

Prostatic part of urethra

Spongy part of urethra [pars cavernosa]

Frena of urethral crest
Urethral crest
Openings of ejaculatory ducts
Openings of prostatic ducts
Membranous part of urethra

Cavity of prostatic utricle

Urethral glands

Corpus spongiosum [corpus cavernosum urethræ]

Fossa terminalis [f. navicularis]

Bladder
Neck of bladder
Prostate
Fascia of sphincter urethræ [fascia diaphragmatis urogenitalis superior]
Bulbo-urethral gland
Perineal membrane [fascia diaphragmatis urogenitalis inferior]
Duct of bulbo-urethral gland
Its orifice
Intrabulbar fossa of urethra

Corpus cavernosum penis : surface which joins with the other in the median plane
Upper wall of urethra
Lower wall of urethra

Valvula fossæ terminalis
Glans penis
External orifice of urethra

PLATE 238.—MALE PERINEUM

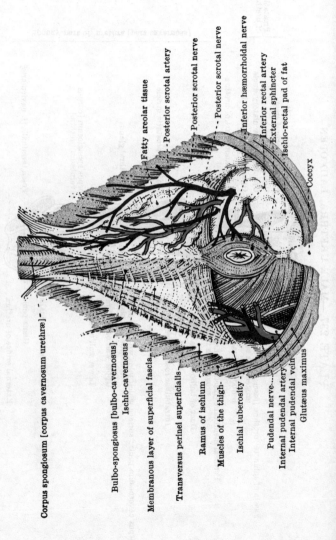

Corpus spongiosum [corpus cavernosum urethrae]

Bulbo-spongiosus [bulbo-cavernosus]
Ischio-cavernosus

Membranous layer of superficial fascia

Transversus perinei superficialis

Ramus of ischium

Muscles of the thigh

Ischial tuberosity

Pudendal nerve
Internal pudendal artery
Internal pudendal vein
Gluteus maximus

Fatty areolar tissue

Posterior scrotal artery

Posterior scrotal nerve

Posterior scrotal nerve

Inferior haemorrhoidal nerve

Inferior rectal artery
External sphincter
Ischio-rectal pad of fat

Coccyx

PLATE 239.—MALE PERINEUM

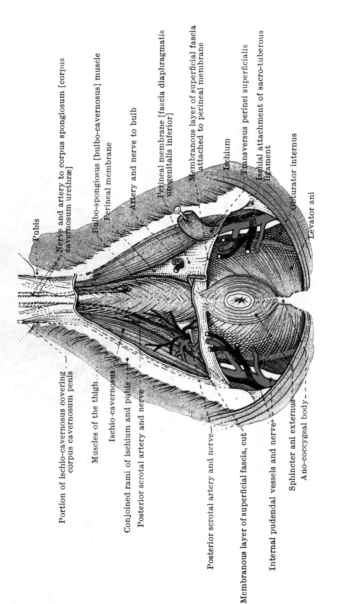

Pubis

Nerve and artery to corpus spongiosum [corpus cavernosum urethræ]

Bulbo-spongiosus [bulbo-cavernosus] muscle

Perineal membrane

Artery and nerve to bulb

Perineal membrane [fascia diaphragmatis urogenitalis inferior]

Membranous layer of superficial fascia attached to perineal membrane

Ischium

Transversus perinei superficialis

Ischial attachment of sacro-tuberous ligament

Obturator internus

Levator ani

Portion of ischio-cavernosus covering corpus cavernosum penis

Muscles of the thigh

Ischio-cavernosus

Conjoined rami of ischium and pubis

Posterior scrotal artery and nerve

Posterior scrotal artery and nerve

Membranous layer of superficial fascia, cut

Internal pudendal vessels and nerve

Sphincter ani externus

Ano-coccygeal body

PLATE 240.—MALE PERINEUM

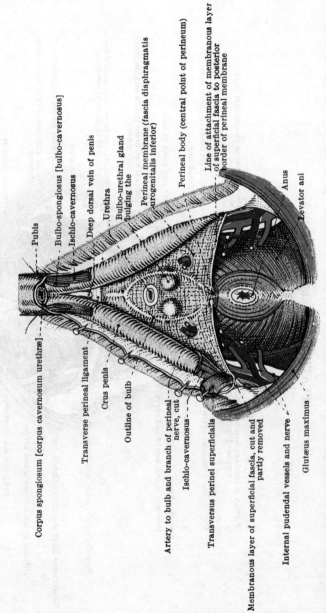

Corpus spongiosum [corpus cavernosum urethræ]

Transverse perineal ligament

Crus penis

Outline of bulb

Artery to bulb and branch of perineal nerve, cut

Ischio-cavernosus

Transversus perinei superficialis

Membranous layer of superficial fascia, cut and partly removed

Internal pudendal vessels and nerve

Glutæus maximus

Pubis

Bulbo-spongiosus [bulbo-cavernosus]

Ischio-cavernosus

Deep dorsal vein of penis

Urethra

Bulbo-urethral gland bulging the

Perineal membrane (fascia diaphragmatis urogenitalis inferior)

Perineal body (central point of perineum)

Line of attachment of membranous layer of superficial fascia to posterior border of perineal membrane

Anus

Levator ani

PLATE 241.—MALE PERINEUM

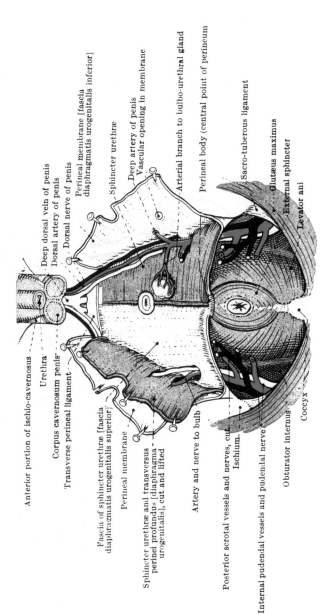

Anterior portion of ischio-cavernosus

Urethra

Corpus cavernosum penis

Transverse perineal ligament

Perineal membrane

Fascia of sphincter urethrae [fascia diaphragmatis urogenitalis superior]

Sphincter urethrae and transversus perinei profundus [diaphragma urogenitalis], cut and lifted

Artery and nerve to bulb

Posterior scrotal vessels and nerves, cut

Ischium

Internal pudendal vessels and pudendal nerve

Obturator internus

Coccyx

Deep dorsal vein of penis

Dorsal artery of penis

Dorsal nerve of penis

Perineal membrane [fascia diaphragmatis urogenitalis inferior]

Sphincter urethrae

Deep artery of penis

Vascular opening in membrane

Arterial branch to bulbo-urethral gland

Perineal body (central point of perineum)

Sacro-tuberous ligament

Gluteus maximus

External sphincter

Levator ani

16

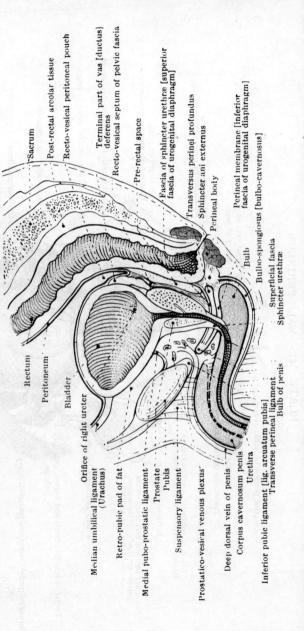

PLATE 242.—MEDIAN SECTION OF MALE PELVIS

Sacrum

Post-rectal areolar tissue

Recto-vesical peritoneal pouch

Terminal part of vas [ductus] deferens

Recto-vesical septum of pelvic fascia

Pre-rectal space

Fascia of sphincter urethræ [superior fascia of urogenital diaphragm]

Transversus perinei profundus

Sphincter ani externus

Perineal body

Perineal membrane [inferior fascia of urogenital diaphragm]

Bulb

Bulbo-spongiosus [bulbo-cavernosus]

Superficial fascia

Sphincter urethræ

Rectum

Peritoneum

Bladder

Orifice of right ureter

Median umbilical ligament (Urachus)

Retro-pubic pad of fat

Medial pubo-prostatic ligament

Prostate

Pubis

Suspensory ligament

Prostatico-vesical venous plexus

Deep dorsal vein of penis

Corpus cavernosum penis

Urethra

Inferior pubic ligament [lig. arcuatum pubis]

Transverse perineal ligament

Bulb of penis

PLATE 243.—SUPERFICIAL AND DEEP RELATIONS OF MALE PERINEUM

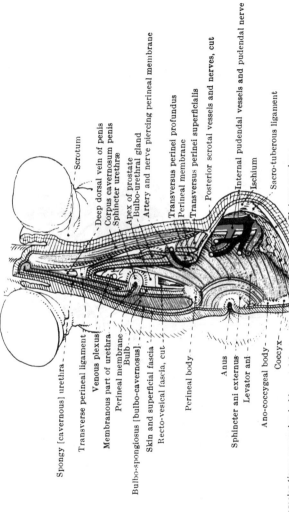

Spongy [cavernous] urethra

Transverse perineal ligament

Venous plexus

Membranous part of urethra

Perineal membrane

Bulb

Bulbo-spongiosus [bulbo-cavernosus]

Skin and superficial fascia

Recto-vesical fascia, cut

Perineal body

Anus

Sphincter ani externus

Levator ani

Ano-coccygeal body

Coccyx

Fatty and areolar tissue occupying ischio-rectal fossa

Scrotum

Deep dorsal vein of penis

Corpus cavernosum penis

Sphincter urethrae

Apex of prostate

Bulbo-urethral gland

Artery and nerve piercing perineal membrane

Transversus perinei profundus

Perineal membrane

Transversus perinei superficialis

Internal pudendal vessels and nerves, cut

Posterior scrotal vessels and nerves, cut

Ischium

Sacro-tuberous ligament

Glutaeus maximus

Skin and superficial fascia

PLATE 244.—VESSELS AND NERVES OF PELVIC CAVITY (MALE)

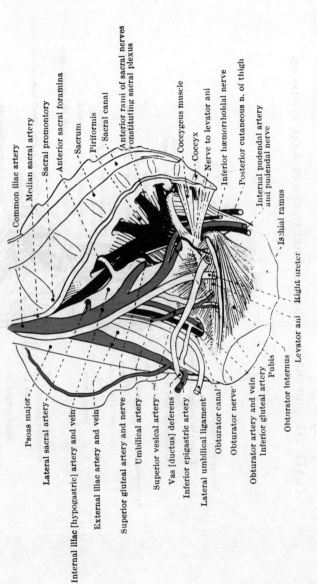

Common iliac artery
Median sacral artery
Sacral promontory
Anterior sacral foramina
Sacrum
Piriformis
Sacral canal
Anterior runni of sacral nerves constituting sacral plexus
Coccygeus muscle
Coccyx
Nerve to levator ani
Inferior hæmorrhoidal nerve
Posterior cutaneous n. of thigh
Internal pudendal artery and pudendal nerve
Ischial ramus
Right ureter

Psoas major
Lateral sacral artery
Internal iliac [hypogastric] artery and vein
External iliac artery and vein
Superior gluteal artery and nerve
Umbilical artery
Superior vesical artery
Vas [ductus] deferens
Inferior epigastric artery
Lateral umbilical ligament
Obturator canal
Obturator nerve
Obturator artery and vein
Inferior gluteal artery
Obturator internus
Pubis
Levator ani

PELVIC COLON RAISED

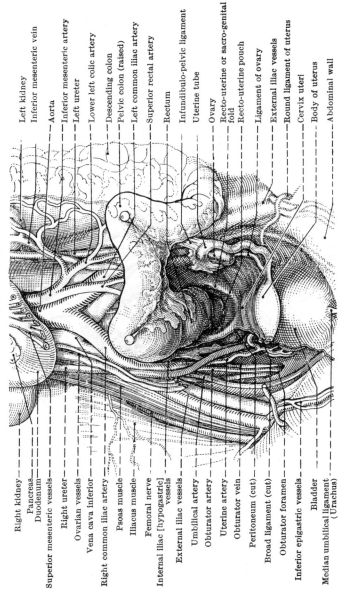

Right kidney
Pancreas
Duodenum
Superior mesenteric vessels
Right ureter
Ovarian vessels
Vena cava inferior
Right common iliac artery
Psoas muscle
Iliacus muscle
Femoral nerve
Internal iliac [hypogastric] vessels
External iliac vessels
Umbilical artery
Obturator artery
Uterine artery
Obturator vein
Peritoneum (cut)
Broad ligament (cut)
Obturator foramen
Inferior epigastric vessels
Bladder
Median umbilical ligament (Urachus)

Left kidney
Inferior mesenteric vein
Aorta
Inferior mesenteric artery
Left ureter
Lower left colic artery
Descending colon
Pelvic colon (raised)
Left common iliac artery
Superior rectal artery
Rectum
Infundibulo-pelvic ligament
Uterine tube
Ovary
Recto-uterine or sacro-genital fold
Recto-uterine pouch
Ligament of ovary
External iliac vessels
Round ligament of uterus
Cervix uteri
Body of uterus
Abdominal wall

PLATE 246.—FEMALE PELVIS

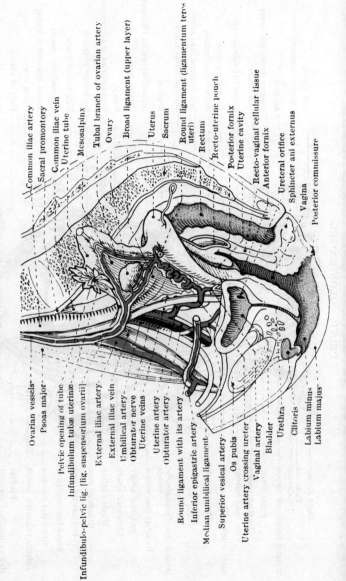

Common iliac artery
Sacral promontory
Common iliac vein
Uterine tube
Mesosalpinx
Tubal branch of ovarian artery
Ovary
Broad ligament (upper layer)
Uterus
Sacrum
Round ligament (ligamentum teres uteri)
Rectum
Recto-uterine pouch
Posterior fornix
Uterine cavity
Recto-vaginal cellular tissue
Anterior fornix
Ureteral orifice
Sphincter ani externus
Vagina
Posterior commissure

Ovarian vessels
Psoas major
Pelvic opening of tube
Infundibulum tubæ uterinæ
Infundibulo-pelvic lig. [lig. suspensorium ovarii]
External iliac artery
External iliac vein
Umbilical artery
Obturator nerve
Uterine veins
Uterine artery
Obturator artery
Round ligament with its artery
Inferior epigastric artery
Median umbilical ligament
Superior vesical artery
Os pubis
Uterine artery crossing ureter
Vaginal artery
Bladder
Urethra
Clitoris
Labium minus
Labium majus

PLATE 247.—FEMALE PELVIS

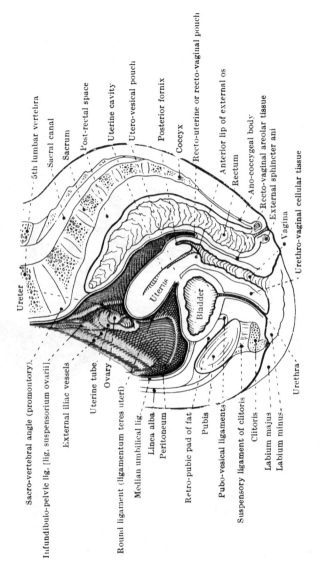

Sacro-vertebral angle (promontory).
Infundibulo-pelvic lig. [lig. suspensorium ovarii]
External iliac vessels
Uterine tube.
Ovary
Round ligament (ligamentum teres uteri)
Median umbilical lig.
Linea alba.
Peritoneum
Retro-pubic pad of fat
Pubis
Pubo-vesical ligaments
Suspensory ligament of clitoris
Clitoris
Labium majus
Labium minus

Ureter

5th lumbar vertebra
Sacral canal
Sacrum
Post-rectal space
Uterine cavity
Utero-vesical pouch
Posterior fornix
Coccyx
Recto-uterine or recto-vaginal pouch
Anterior lip of external os
Rectum
Ano-coccygeal body
Recto-vaginal areolar tissue
External sphincter ani
Vagina
Urethro-vaginal cellular tissue

Uterus

Bladder

Urethra

PLATE 248.—FEMALE PERINEUM

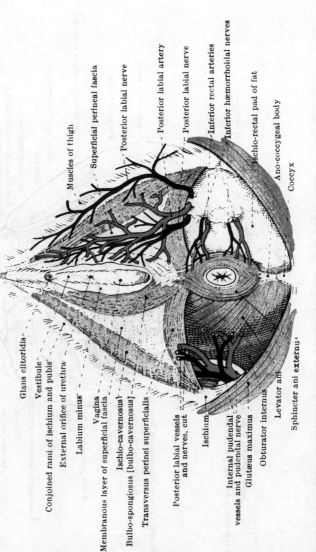

Glans clitoridis
Vestibule
Conjoined rami of ischium and pubis
External orifice of urethra
Labium minus
Vagina
Membranous layer of superficial fascia
Ischio-cavernosus¹
Bulbo-spongiosus [bulbo-cavernosus]
Transversus perinei superficialis
Posterior labial vessels and nerves, cut
Internal pudendal vessels and pudendal nerve
Gluteus maximus
Obturator internus
Ischium
Levator ani
Sphincter ani externu²

Muscles of thigh
Superficial perineal fascia
Posterior labial nerve
Posterior labial artery
Posterior labial nerve
Inferior rectal arteries
Inferior hæmorrhoital nerves
Ischio-rectal pad of fat
Ano-coccygeal body
Coccyx

PLATE 249.—FEMALE PERINEUM

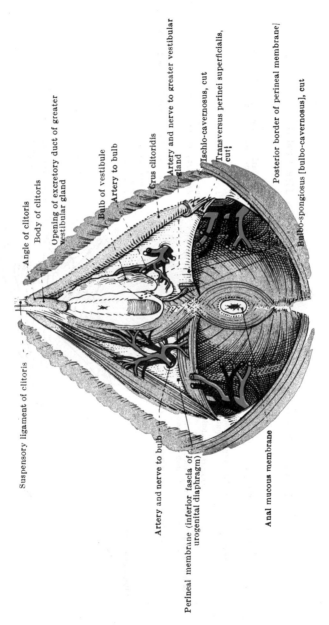

Suspensory ligament of clitoris

Angle of clitoris

Body of clitoris

Opening of excretory duct of greater vestibular gland

Bulb of vestibule

Artery to bulb

Crus clitoridis

Artery and nerve to greater vestibular gland

Ischio-cavernosus, cut

Transversus perinei superficialis, cut

Posterior border of perineal membrane

Bulbo-spongiosus [bulbo-cavernosus], cut

Anal mucous membrane

Artery and nerve to bulb

Perineal membrane (inferior fascia of urogenital diaphragm)

PLATE 250.—LEVATOR ANI—UPPER ASPECT—IN THE FEMALE

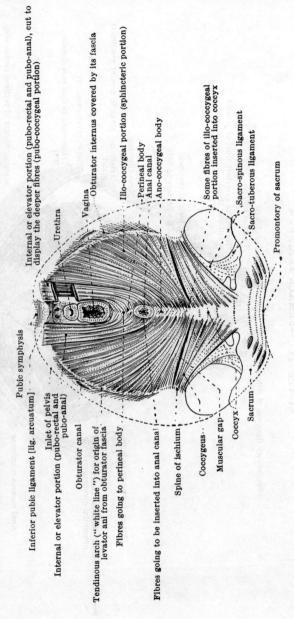

Pubic symphysis

Inferior pubic ligament [lig. arcuatum]

Inlet of pelvis

Internal or elevator portion (pubo-rectal and pubo-anal)

Obturator canal

Tendinous arch ("white line") for origin of levator ani from obturator fascia

Fibres going to perineal body

Fibres going to be inserted into anal canal

Spine of ischium

Coccygeus

Muscular gap

Coccyx

Sacrum

Internal or elevator portion (pubo-rectal and pubo-anal), cut to display the deeper fibres (pubo-coccygeal portion)

Urethra

Vagina

Obturator internus covered by its fascia

Illo-coccygeal portion (sphincteric portion)

Perineal body

Anal canal

Ano-coccygeal body

Some fibres of ilio-coccygeal portion inserted into coccyx

Sacro-spinous ligament

Sacro-tuberous ligament

Promontory of sacrum

PLATE 251.—CORONAL SECTION THROUGH UTERUS AND VAGINA

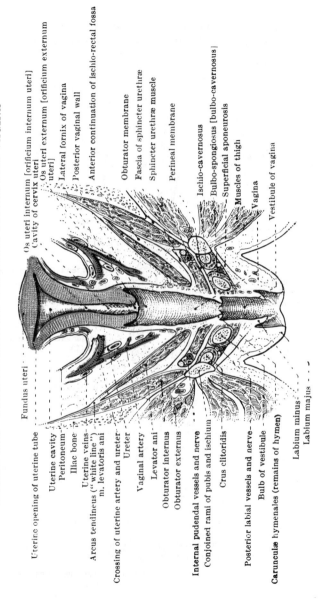

Os uteri internum [orificium internum uteri]
Cavity of cervix uteri
Os uteri externum [orificium externum uteri]
Lateral fornix of vagina
Posterior vaginal wall
Anterior continuation of ischio-rectal fossa

Obturator membrane
Fascia of sphincter urethræ
Sphincter urethræ muscle
Perineal membrane

Ischio-cavernosus
Bulbo-spongiosus [bulbo-cavernosus]
Superficial aponeurosis
Muscles of thigh
Vagina
Vestibule of vagina

Fundus uteri

Uterine opening of uterine tube
Uterine cavity
Peritoneum
Iliac bone
Uterine veins ("white line")
Arcus tendineus m. levatoris ani

Crossing of uterine artery and ureter
Ureter
Vaginal artery
Levator ani
Obturator internus
Obturator externus

Internal pudendal vessels and nerve
Conjoined rami of pubis and ischium
Crus clitoridis

Posterior labial vessels and nerve
Bulb of vestibule
Carunculæ hymenales (remains of hymen)

Labium minus
Labium majus

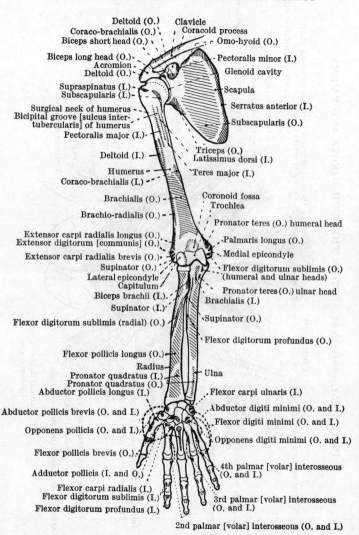

Deltoid (O.)
Coraco-brachialis (O.)
Biceps short head (O.)
Clavicle
Coracoid process
Omo-hyoid (O.)

Biceps long head (O.)
Acromion
Deltoid (O.)
Pectoralis minor (I.)
Glenoid cavity

Supraspinatus (I.)
Subscapularis (I.)
Scapula
Serratus anterior (I.)

Surgical neck of humerus
Bicipital groove [sulcus inter-tubercularis] of humerus
Pectoralis major (I.)
Subscapularis (O.)

Deltoid (I.)
Triceps (O.)
Latissimus dorsi (I.)

Humerus
Coraco-brachialis (I.)
Teres major (I.)

Brachialis (O.)
Coronoid fossa
Trochlea

Brachio-radialis (O.)
Pronator teres (O.) humeral head

Extensor carpi radialis longus (O.)
Extensor digitorum [communis] (O.)
Palmaris longus (O.)

Extensor carpi radialis brevis (O.)
Medial epicondyle

Supinator (O.)
Lateral epicondyle
Capitulum
Flexor digitorum sublimis (O.) (humeral and ulnar heads)

Biceps brachii (I.)
Pronator teres (O.) ulnar head
Brachialis (I.)

Supinator (I.)
Supinator (O.)

Flexor digitorum sublimis (radial) (O.)
Flexor digitorum profundus (O.)

Flexor pollicis longus (O.)
Radius
Pronator quadratus (I.)
Pronator quadratus (O.)
Abductor pollicis longus (I.)
Ulna
Flexor carpi ulnaris (I.)

Abductor pollicis brevis (O. and I.)
Abductor digiti minimi (O. and I.)

Opponens pollicis (O. and I.)
Flexor digiti minimi (O. and I.)
Opponens digiti minimi (O. and I.)

Flexor pollicis brevis (O.)

Adductor pollicis (I. and O.)
4th palmar [volar] interosseous (O. and I.)

Flexor carpi radialis (I.)
Flexor digitorum sublimis (I.)
Flexor digitorum profundus (I.)
3rd palmar [volar] interosseous (O. and I.)

2nd palmar [volar] interosseous (O. and I.)

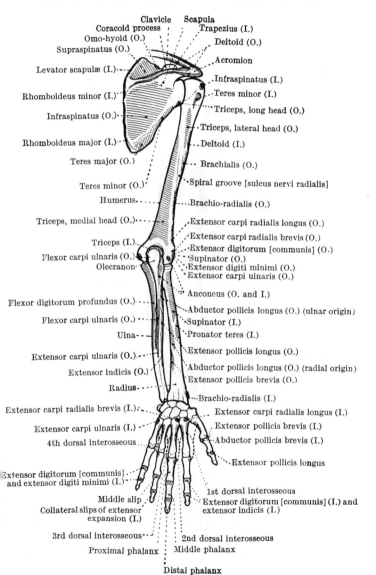

Clavicle
Scapula

Coracoid process
Trapezius (I.)

Omo-hyoid (O.)
Deltoid (O.)

Supraspinatus (O.)

Levator scapulæ (I.)
Acromion

Infraspinatus (I.)

Rhomboideus minor (I.)
Teres minor (I.)

Triceps, long head (O.)

Infraspinatus (O.)
Triceps, lateral head (O.)

Deltoid (I.)

Rhomboideus major (I.)
Brachialis (O.)

Teres major (O.)

Teres minor (O.)
Spiral groove [sulcus nervi radialis]

Humerus
Brachio-radialis (O.)

Triceps, medial head (O.)
Extensor carpi radialis longus (O.)

Extensor carpi radialis brevis (O.)

Triceps (I.)
Extensor digitorum [communis] (O.)

Supinator (O.)

Flexor carpi ulnaris (O.)
Extensor digiti minimi (O.)

Olecranon
Extensor carpi ulnaris (O.)

Anconeus (O. and I.)

Flexor digitorum profundus (O.)
Abductor pollicis longus (O.) (ulnar origin)

Flexor carpi ulnaris (O.)
Supinator (I.)

Ulna
Pronator teres (I.)

Extensor carpi ulnaris (O.)
Extensor pollicis longus (O.)

Extensor indicis (O.)
Abductor pollicis longus (O.) (radial origin)

Extensor pollicis brevis (O.)

Radius
Brachio-radialis (I.)

Extensor carpi radialis brevis (I.)
Extensor carpi radialis longus (I.)

Extensor carpi ulnaris (I.)
Extensor pollicis brevis (I.)

4th dorsal interosseous
Abductor pollicis brevis (I.)

Extensor pollicis longus

Extensor digitorum [communis]
and extensor digiti minimi (I.)

1st dorsal interosseous

Middle slip
Extensor digitorum [communis] (I.) and
extensor indicis (I.)

Collateral slips of extensor
expansion (I.)

3rd dorsal interosseous
2nd dorsal interosseous

Proximal phalanx
Middle phalanx

Distal phalanx

PLATE 254.—MUSCLES OF UPPER LIMB
ANTERIOR ASPECT

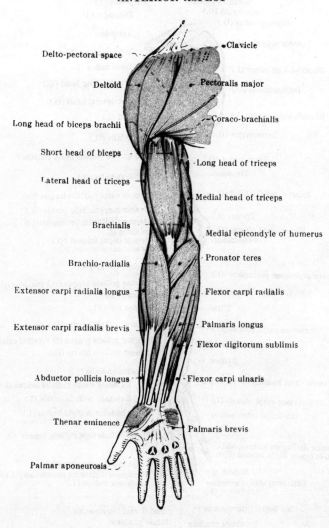

Delto-pectoral space

Deltoid

Long head of biceps brachii

Short head of biceps

Lateral head of triceps

Brachialis

Brachio-radialis

Extensor carpi radialis longus

Extensor carpi radialis brevis

Abductor pollicis longus

Thenar eminence

Palmar aponeurosis

Clavicle

Pectoralis major

Coraco-brachialis

Long head of triceps

Medial head of triceps

Medial epicondyle of humerus

Pronator teres

Flexor carpi radialis

Palmaris longus

Flexor digitorum sublimis

Flexor carpi ulnaris

Palmaris brevis

PLATE 255.—MUSCLES OF UPPER LIMB
POSTERIOR ASPECT

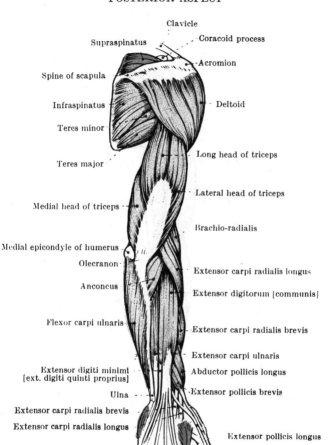

Clavicle

Coracoid process

Supraspinatus

Acromion

Spine of scapula

Infraspinatus

Deltoid

Teres minor

Long head of triceps

Teres major

Lateral head of triceps

Medial head of triceps

Brachio-radialis

Medial epicondyle of humerus

Olecranon

Extensor carpi radialis longus

Anconeus

Extensor digitorum [communis]

Flexor carpi ulnaris

Extensor carpi radialis brevis

Extensor carpi ulnaris

Extensor digiti minimi
[ext. digiti quinti proprius]

Abductor pollicis longus

Ulna

Extensor pollicis brevis

Extensor carpi radialis brevis

Extensor carpi radialis longus

Extensor pollicis longus

PLATE 256.—MUSCLES OF UPPER LIMB
MEDIAL ASPECT

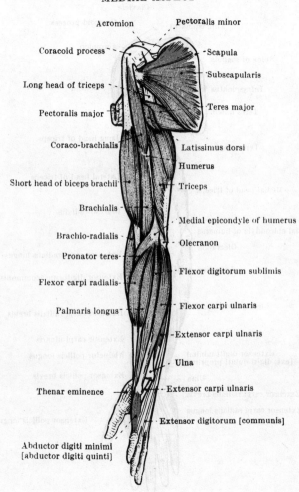

Acromion

Pectoralis minor

Coracoid process

Scapula

Long head of triceps

Subscapularis

Pectoralis major

Teres major

Coraco-brachialis

Latissimus dorsi

Humerus

Short head of biceps brachii

Triceps

Brachialis

Medial epicondyle of humerus

Brachio-radialis

Olecranon

Pronator teres

Flexor digitorum sublimis

Flexor carpi radialis

Flexor carpi ulnaris

Palmaris longus

Extensor carpi ulnaris

Ulna

Thenar eminence

Extensor carpi ulnaris

Extensor digitorum [communis]

Abductor digiti minimi
[abductor digiti quinti]

PLATE 257.—MUSCLES OF UPPER LIMB
LATERAL ASPECT

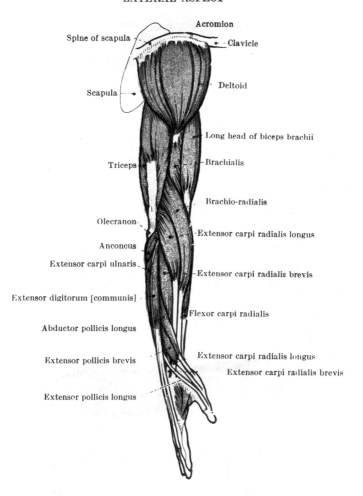

Acromion

Spine of scapula

Clavicle

Deltoid

Scapula

Long head of biceps brachii

Brachialis

Triceps

Brachio-radialis

Olecranon

Extensor carpi radialis longus

Anconeus

Extensor carpi ulnaris

Extensor carpi radialis brevis

Extensor digitorum [communis]

Flexor carpi radialis

Abductor pollicis longus

Extensor pollicis brevis

Extensor carpi radialis longus

Extensor carpi radialis brevis

Extensor pollicis longus

PLATE 258.—MUSCLES ON FRONT AND BACK OF UPPER ARM

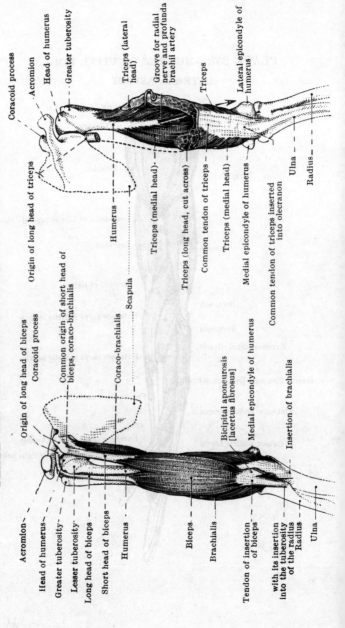

Acromion
Head of humerus
Greater tuberosity
Lesser tuberosity
Long head of biceps
Short head of biceps
Humerus

Biceps
Brachialis

Tendon of insertion of biceps

with its insertion into the tuberosity of the radius
Radius
Ulna

Origin of long head of biceps
Coracoid process
Common origin of short head of biceps, coraco-brachialis

Coraco-brachialis
Scapula

Bicipital aponeurosis [lacertus fibrosus]
Medial epicondyle of humerus

Insertion of brachialis

Coracoid process
Acromion
Head of humerus
Greater tuberosity

Origin of long head of triceps

Humerus

Triceps (medial head)

Triceps (lateral head)
Groove for radial nerve and profunda brachii artery
Triceps
Lateral epicondyle of humerus

Triceps (long head, cut across)
Common tendon of triceps
Triceps (medial head)
Medial epicondyle of humerus

Common tendon of triceps inserted into olecranon

Ulna
Radius

PLATE 259.—MUSCLES OF THE FOREARM—ANTERIOR ASPECT

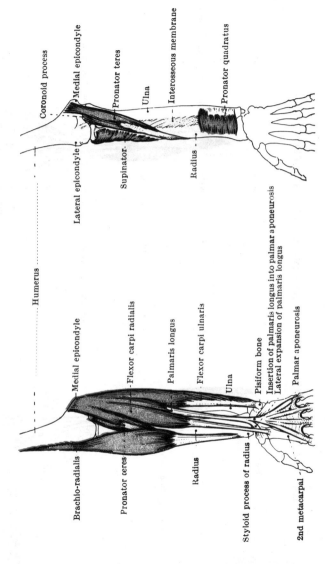

Coronoid process

Medial epicondyle

Pronator teres

Ulna

Interosseous membrane

Pronator quadratus

Lateral epicondyle

Supinator

Radius

Humerus

Medial epicondyle

Flexor carpi radialis

Palmaris longus

Flexor carpi ulnaris

Ulna

Pisiform bone

Insertion of palmaris longus into palmar aponeurosis
Lateral expansion of palmaris longus

Palmar aponeurosis

Brachio-radialis

Pronator ceres

Radius

Styloid process of radius

2nd metacarpal

PLATE 260.—MUSCLES OF THE FOREARM—ANTERIOR ASPECT (*Continued*)

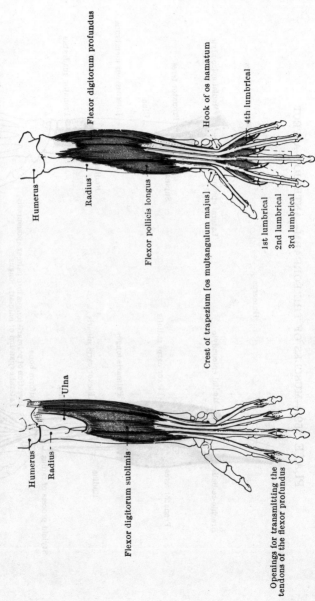

Humerus

Radius

Flexor digitorum profundus

Radius

Flexor pollicis longus

Hook of os hamatum

4th lumbrical

Crest of trapezium [os multangulum majus]

1st lumbrical

2nd lumbrical

3rd lumbrical

Humerus

Ulna

Radius

Flexor digitorum sublimis

Openings for transmitting the
tendons of the flexor profundus

PLATE 261.—MUSCLES OF THE FOREARM—POSTERIOR ASPECT

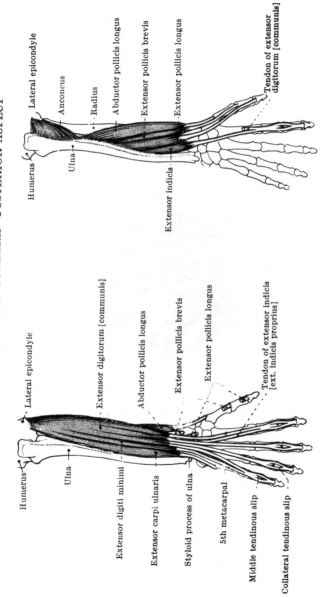

PLATE 262.—MUSCLES OF HAND—PALMAR [VOLAR] ASPECT

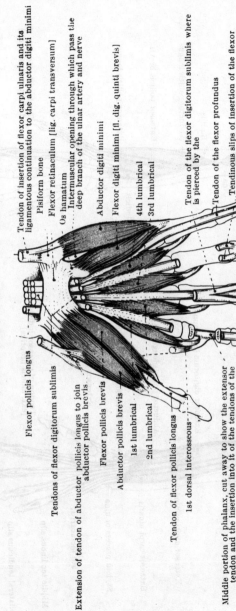

Flexor pollicis longus

Tendons of flexor digitorum sublimis

Extension of tendon of abductor pollicis longus to join
abductor pollicis brevis

Flexor pollicis brevis

1st lumbrical

2nd lumbrical

Tendon of flexor pollicis longus

1st dorsal interosseous

Middle portion of phalanx, cut away to show the extensor
tendon and the insertion into it of the tendons of the
short muscles

Tendon of insertion of flexor carpi ulnaris and its
ligamentous continuation to the abductor digiti minimi

Pisiform bone

Flexor retinaculum [lig. carpi transversum]

Os hamatum

Internuscular opening through which pass the
deep branch of the ulnar artery and nerve

Abductor digiti minimi

Flexor digiti minimi [fl. dig. quinti brevis]

4th lumbrical

3rd lumbrical

Tendon of the flexor digitorum sublimis where
is pierced by the

Tendon of the flexor profundus

Tendinous slips of insertion of the flexor
digitorum sublimis

Insertion of tendon of flexor digitorum
profundus

Abductor pollicis brevis

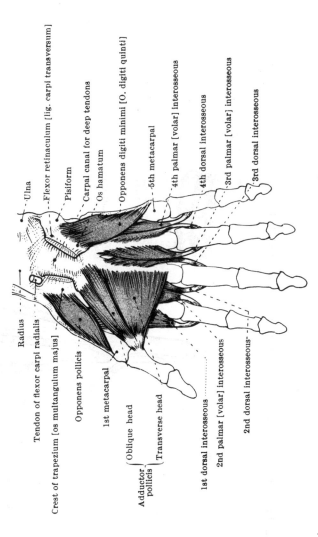

PLATE 263.—MUSCLES OF THE HAND (*Continued*)

Radius

Tendon of flexor carpi radialis

Crest of trapezium [os multangulum majus]

Opponens pollicis

1st metacarpal

Adductor pollicis { Oblique head
Transverse head }

1st dorsal interosseous

2nd palmar [volar] interosseous

2nd dorsal interosseous

Ulna

Flexor retinaculum [lig. carpi transversum]

Pisiform

Carpal canal for deep tendons

Os hamatum

Opponens digiti minimi [O. digiti quinti]

5th metacarpal

4th palmar [volar] interosseous

4th dorsal interosseous

3rd palmar [volar] interosseous

3rd dorsal interosseous

PLATE 264.—SYNOVIAL TENDON SHEATHS OF PALMAR [VOLAR] ASPECT OF HAND

Vincula connecting tendons of flexor digitorum sublimis and flexor digitorum profundus

Visceral layer of synovial sheath

Intertendinous synovial space

Parietal layer of synovial sheath

Tendons of flexor digitorum sublimis and flexor digitorum profundus

Common sheath of superficial and deep flexor tendons of the fingers

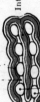

Tendons of flexor digitorum profundus

Tendons of flexor digitorum sublimis

Tendon of flexor pollicis longus

Tendon sheath of flexor pollicis longus

Digital synovial sheaths of { index finger · middle finger · ring finger · ·

Insertions of tendons (perforating) of flexor digitorum profundus

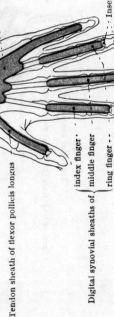

PLATE 265.—SYNOVIAL TENDON SHEATHS OF BACK OF HAND

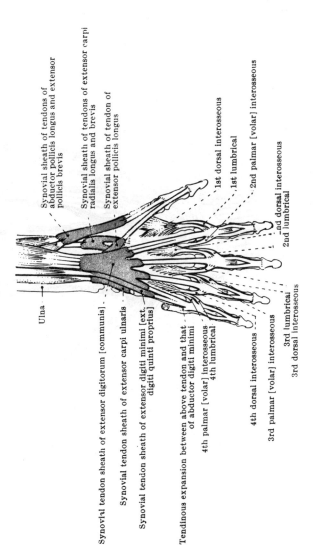

Synovial sheath of tendons of abductor pollicis longus and extensor pollicis brevis

Synovial sheath of tendons of extensor carpi radialis longus and brevis

Synovial sheath of tendon of extensor pollicis longus

1st dorsal interosseous

1st lumbrical

2nd palmar [volar] interosseous

2nd dorsal interosseous

2nd lumbrical

Ulna

Synovial tendon sheath of extensor digitorum [communis]

Synovial tendon sheath of extensor carpi ulnaris

Synovial tendon sheath of extensor digiti minimi [ext. digiti quinti proprius]

Tendinous expansion between above tendon and that of abductor digiti minimi

4th palmar [volar] interosseous

4th lumbrical

4th dorsal interosseous

3rd lumbrical

3rd palmar [volar] interosseous

3rd dorsal interosseous

PLATE 266.—VESSELS AND NERVES OF THE HAND—PALMAR [VOLAR] ASPECT

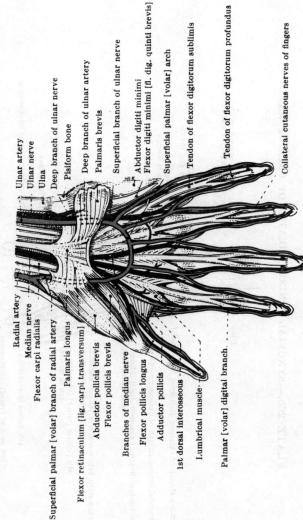

Radial artery
Median nerve
Flexor carpi radialis
Superficial palmar [volar] branch of radial artery
Palmaris longus
Flexor retinaculum [lig. carpi transversum]
Abductor pollicis brevis
Flexor pollicis brevis
Branches of median nerve
Flexor pollicis longus
Adductor pollicis
1st dorsal interosseous
Lumbrical muscle
Palmar [volar] digital branch.

Ulnar artery
Ulnar nerve
Ulna
Deep branch of ulnar nerve
Pisiform bone
Deep branch of ulnar artery
Palmaris brevis
Superficial branch of ulnar nerve
Abductor digiti minimi
Flexor digiti minimi [fl. dig. quinti brevis]
Superficial palmar [volar] arch
Tendon of flexor digitorum sublimis
Tendon of flexor digitorum profundus
Collateral cutaneous nerves of fingers

PLATE 267.—VESSELS AND NERVES OF THE HAND—PALMAR [VOLAR] ASPECT—
DEEP DISSECTION

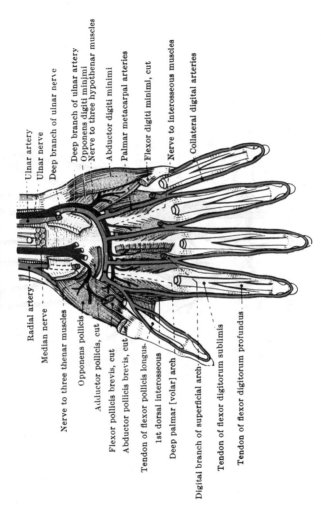

Radial artery
Median nerve
Nerve to three thenar muscles
Opponens pollicis
Flexor pollicis brevis, cut
Abductor pollicis brevis, cut
Tendon of flexor pollicis longus
1st dorsal interosseous
Deep palmar [volar] arch
Digital branch of superficial arch
Tendon of flexor digitorum sublimis
Tendon of flexor digitorum profundus

Ulnar artery
Ulnar nerve
Deep branch of ulnar nerve
Deep branch of ulnar artery
Opponens digiti minimi
Nerve to three hypothenar muscles
Abductor digiti minimi
Palmar metacarpal arteries
Flexor digiti minimi, cut
Nerve to interosseous muscles
Collateral digital arteries

PLATE 268.—ARTERIES OF THE HAND—PALMAR [VOLAR] ASPECT

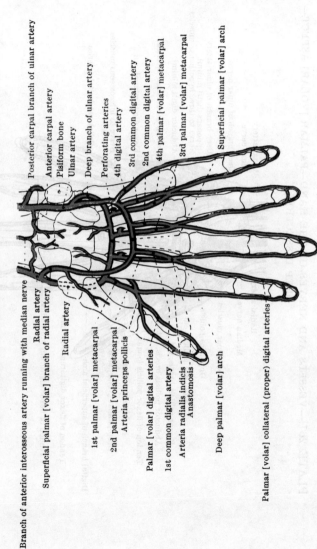

Branch of anterior interosseous artery running with median nerve

Radial artery

Superficial palmar [volar] branch of radial artery

Radial artery

1st palmar [volar] metacarpal

2nd palmar [volar] metacarpal
Arteria princeps pollicis

Palmar [volar] digital arteries

1st common digital artery

Arteria radialis indicis
Anastomosis

Deep palmar [volar] arch

Palmar [volar] collateral (proper) digital arteries

Posterior carpal branch of ulnar artery

Anterior carpal artery

Pisiform bone

Ulnar artery

Deep branch of ulnar artery

Perforating arteries

4th digital artery

3rd common digital artery

2nd common digital artery

4th palmar [volar] metacarpal

3rd palmar [volar] metacarpal

Superficial palmar [volar] arch

PLATE 269.—ARTERIES OF THE HAND—DORSAL ASPECT

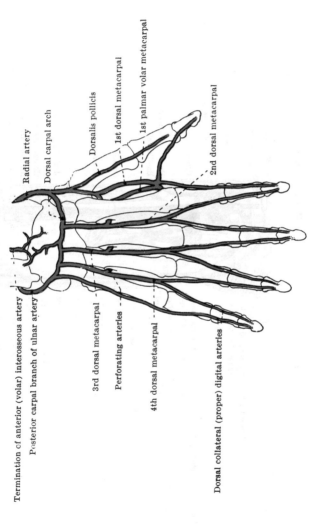

Termination of anterior (volar) interosseous artery

Posterior carpal branch of ulnar artery

Radial artery

Dorsal carpal arch

Dorsalis pollicis

1st dorsal metacarpal

1st palmar volar metacarpal

2nd dorsal metacarpal

3rd dorsal metacarpal

Perforating arteries

4th dorsal metacarpal

Dorsal collateral (proper) digital arteries

PLATE 270.—UPPER ARM—ANTERIOR ASPECT

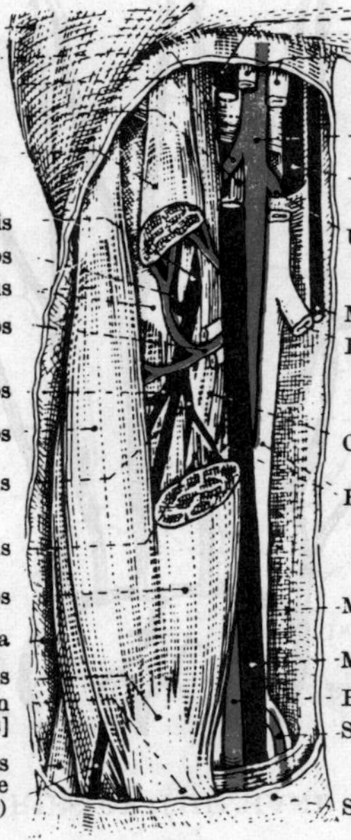

Median nerve
Basilic vein
Pectoralis major
Brachial artery
Ulnar nerve passing behind intermuscular septum
Ulnar collateral artery
Medial cutaneous nerve of forearm
Basilic vein
Coraco-brachialis muscle
Brachial veins
Medial intermuscular septum
Median nerve
Brachial artery
Supratrochlear artery [a. collateralis ulnaris inferior]
Superficial fascia

Deltoid
Teres major
Posterior humeral circumflex art.
Long head of triceps
Short head of biceps
Musculo-cutaneous nerve after piercing coraco-brachialis
Nerve to short head of biceps
Humerus
Artery to biceps
Nerve to long head of biceps
Long head of biceps
Nerve to brachialis
Brachialis
Short head of biceps
Superficial fascia
Tendon of biceps
Its aponeurotic expansion [lacertus fibrosus]
Brachio-radialis
Cutaneous branch of musculo-cutaneous nerve (lateral cutaneous nerve of forearm)

PLATE 271.—UPPER ARM—POSTERIOR ASPECT

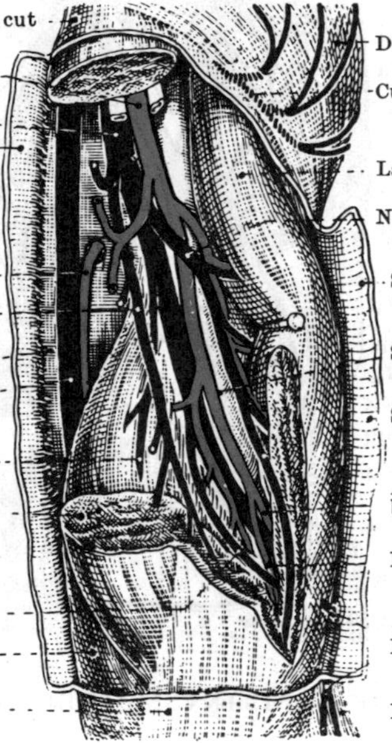

Long head of triceps, cut

Deltoid

Cutaneous branches of the circumflex [axillary] nerve

Profunda brachii artery

Radial nerve

Superficial fascia

Lateral head of triceps

Nerve to lateral head of triceps and anconeus

Superficial fascia

Ulnar collateral artery

Spiral groove [sulcus nervi radialis]

Nerve to long head of triceps

Superficial fascia

Medial intermuscular septum

Ulnar nerve

Anterior terminal branch of superior profunda brachii artery

Nerve to triceps

Its posterior terminal branch

Long head of triceps, cut

Radial nerve [ramus superficialis]

Radial nerve

Portion of triceps

Brachio-radialis

Triceps

PLATE 272.—ELBOW—ANTERIOR ASPECT

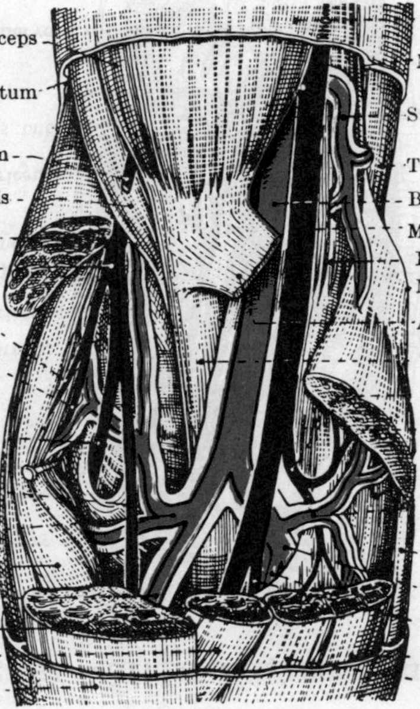

Biceps

Lateral intermuscular septum

Lateral cutaneous nerve of forearm

Brachialis
Brachio-radialis, cut
Radial nerve

Nerve to extensor carpi radialis longus

Nerve to extensor carpi radialis brevis

Posterior interosseous nerve (motor) [ramus
profundus nervi radialis] piercing supinator

Radial nerve (sensory) [ramus
superficialis nervi radialis]

Radial recurrent artery

Extensor carpi radialis longus

Radial artery
Brachio-radialis, cut
Pronator teres
Superficial fascia

Superficial fascia

Medial intermuscular septum

Supratrochlear artery [a. collateralis ulnaris inferior]

Triceps

Brachial artery

Median nerve

Brachialis

Medial epicondyle

Aponeurotic expansion of biceps
tendon [lacertus fibrosus]

Tendon of biceps

Muscular branches of nerves

Flexor muscles arising from epicondyle, cut

Flexor digitorum profundus

Common trunk of posterior and anterior
ulnar recurrent branches

Flexor carpi ulnaris

Ulnar artery

Common interosseous artery and nerve

Palmaris longus, cut
Flexor carpi radialis, cut

PLATE 273.—ELBOW—POSTERIOR ASPECT

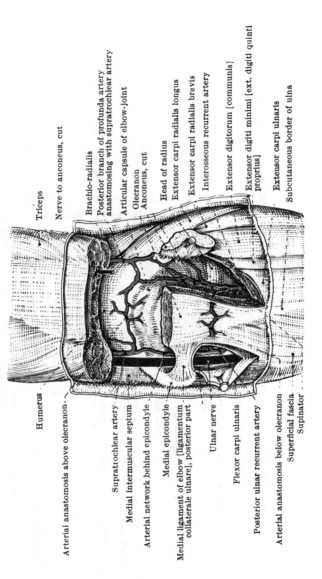

Triceps

Nerve to anconeus, cut

Brachio-radialis

Posterior branch of profunda artery anastomosing with supratrochlear artery

Articular capsule of elbow-joint

Olecranon

Anconeus, cut

Head of radius

Extensor carpi radialis longus

Extensor carpi radialis brevis

Interosseous recurrent artery

Extensor digitorum [communis]

Extensor digiti minimi [ext. digiti quinti proprius]

Extensor carpi ulnaris

Subcutaneous border of ulna

Humerus

Arterial anastomosis above olecranon

Supratrochlear artery

Medial intermuscular septum

Arterial network behind epicondyle

Medial epicondyle

Medial ligament of elbow [ligamentum collaterale ulnare], posterior part

Ulnar nerve

Flexor carpi ulnaris

Posterior ulnar recurrent artery

Arterial anastomosis below olecranon

Superficial fascia

Supinator

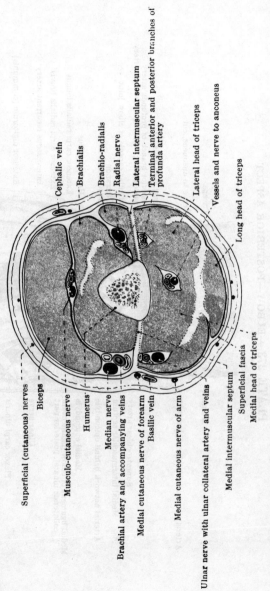

PLATE 274.—TRANSVERSE SECTION THROUGH MIDDLE OF UPPER ARM

Superficial (cutaneous) nerves
Biceps
Musculo-cutaneous nerve
Humerus
Median nerve
Brachial artery and accompanying veins
Medial cutaneous nerve of forearm
Basilic vein
Medial cutaneous nerve of arm
Ulnar nerve with ulnar collateral artery and veins
Medial intermuscular septum
Superficial fascia
Medial head of triceps

Cephalic vein
Brachialis
Brachio-radialis
Radial nerve
Lateral intermuscular septum
Terminal anterior and posterior branches of profunda artery
Lateral head of triceps
Vessels and nerve to anconeus
Long head of triceps

PLATE 275.—TRANSVERSE SECTION AT LEVEL OF ELBOW

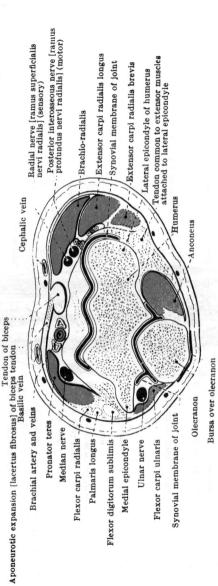

Aponeurotic expansion [lacertus fibrosus] of biceps tendon
Tendon of biceps
Basilic vein
Cephalic vein
Brachial artery and veins
Pronator teres
Median nerve
Flexor carpi radialis
Palmaris longus
Flexor digitorum sublimis
Medial epicondyle
Ulnar nerve
Flexor carpi ulnaris
Synovial membrane of joint
Olecranon
Bursa over olecranon

Radial nerve [ramus superficialis nervi radialis] (sensory)
Posterior interosseous nerve [ramus profundus nervi radialis] (motor)
Brachio-radialis
Extensor carpi radialis longus
Synovial membrane of joint
Extensor carpi radialis brevis
Lateral epicondyle of humerus
Tendon common to extensor muscles attached to lateral epicondyle
Humerus
Anconeus

PLATE 276.—FOREARM—ANTERIOR ASPECT

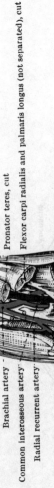

Brachial artery
Common interosseous artery
Radial recurrent artery

Flexor digitorum profundus

Pronator teres, cut
Brachio-radialis
Extensor carpi radialis longus
Flexor pollicis longus
Extensor carpi radialis brevis

Radial nerve [ramus superficialis] (sensory)
Radial artery
Interosseous membrane
Median nerve
Radius
Pronator quadratus
Flexor carpi radialis

Pronator teres, cut
Flexor carpi radialis and palmaris longus (not separated), cut

Flexor digitorum sublimis, cut

Ulnar nerve
Ulnar artery
Flexor carpi ulnaris
Flexor digitorum profundus

Anterior interosseous artery and nerve

Tendons of the flexor digitorum sublimis, cut

Tendon of palmaris longus

PLATE 277.—FOREARM—POSTERIOR ASPECT

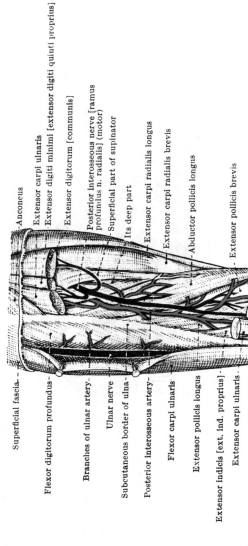

Superficial fascia

Anconeus

Extensor carpi ulnaris

Extensor digiti minimi [extensor digiti quinti proprius]

Extensor digitorum [communis]

Flexor digitorum profundus

Posterior interosseous nerve [ramus profundus n. radialis] (motor)

Superficial part of supinator

Its deep part

Branches of ulnar artery

Ulnar nerve

Subcutaneous border of ulna

Extensor carpi radialis longus

Extensor carpi radialis brevis

Posterior interosseous artery

Abductor pollicis longus

Flexor carpi ulnaris

Extensor pollicis longus

Extensor pollicis brevis

Extensor indicis [ext. ind. proprius]

Extensor digiti minimi [ext. digiti quinti proprius]

Extensor digitorum [communis]

Superficial fascia

PLATE 278.—SECTION THROUGH MIDDLE OF FOREARM

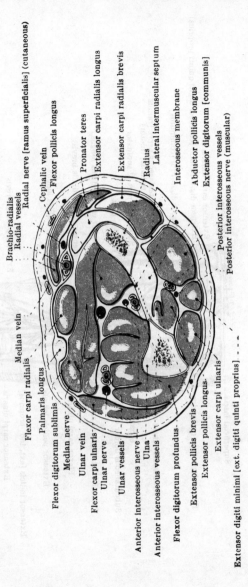

PLATE 279.—SECTION THROUGH FOREARM A LITTLE ABOVE WRIST

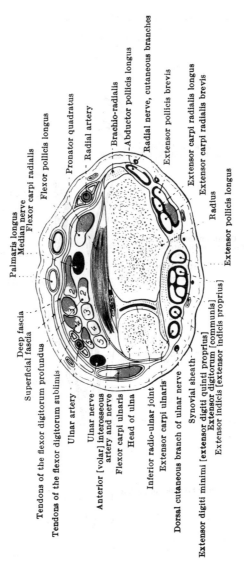

PLATE 280.—CUTANEOUS NERVES OF UPPER LIMB
ANTERIOR ASPECT

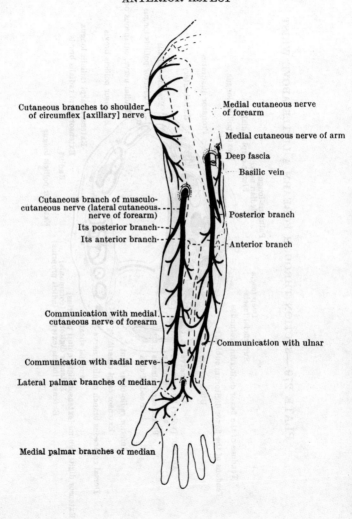

Cutaneous branches to shoulder
of circumflex [axillary] nerve

Medial cutaneous nerve
of forearm

Medial cutaneous nerve of arm

Deep fascia

Basilic vein

Cutaneous branch of musculo-
cutaneous nerve (lateral cutaneous
nerve of forearm)

Its posterior branch

Its anterior branch

Posterior branch

Anterior branch

Communication with medial
cutaneous nerve of forearm

Communication with ulnar

Communication with radial nerve

Lateral palmar branches of median

Medial palmar branches of median

PLATE 281.—CUTANEOUS NERVES OF UPPER LIMB
POSTERIOR ASPECT

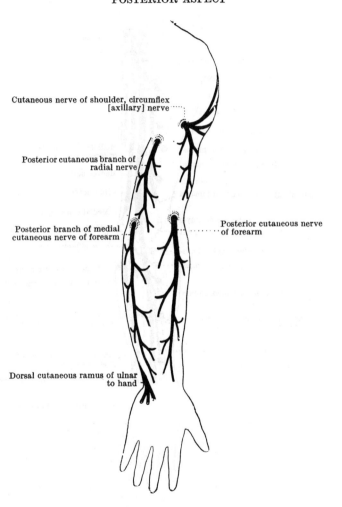

Cutaneous nerve of shoulder, circumflex [axillary] nerve

Posterior cutaneous branch of radial nerve

Posterior branch of medial cutaneous nerve of forearm

Posterior cutaneous nerve of forearm

Dorsal cutaneous ramus of ulnar to hand

PLATE 282.—MUSCULAR NERVES OF UPPER LIMB
ANTERIOR ASPECT

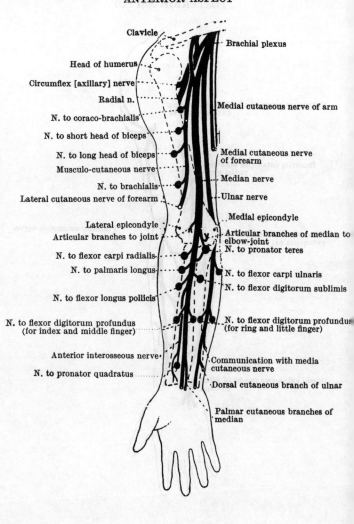

Clavicle

Brachial plexus

Head of humerus

Circumflex [axillary] nerve

Radial n.

N. to coraco-brachialis

N. to short head of biceps

N. to long head of biceps

Musculo-cutaneous nerve

N. to brachialis

Lateral cutaneous nerve of forearm

Lateral epicondyle

Articular branches to joint

N. to flexor carpi radialis

N. to palmaris longus

N. to flexor longus pollicis

N. to flexor digitorum profundus
(for index and middle finger)

Anterior interosseous nerve

N. to pronator quadratus

Medial cutaneous nerve of arm

Medial cutaneous nerve
of forearm

Median nerve

Ulnar nerve

Medial epicondyle

Articular branches of median to
elbow-joint

N. to pronator teres

N. to flexor carpi ulnaris

N. to flexor digitorum sublimis

N. to flexor digitorum profundus
(for ring and little finger)

Communication with media
cutaneous nerve

Dorsal cutaneous branch of ulnar

Palmar cutaneous branches of
median

PLATE 283.—MUSCULAR NERVES OF UPPER LIMB
POSTERIOR ASPECT

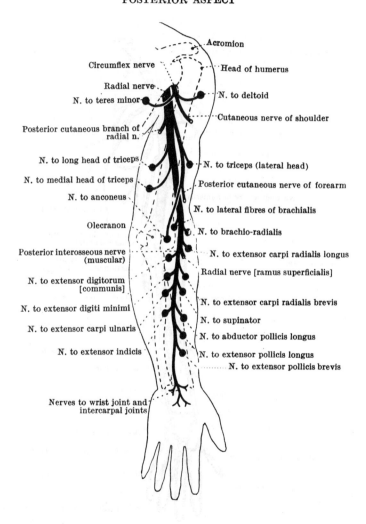

Acromion

Circumflex nerve

Head of humerus

Radial nerve

N. to teres minor

N. to deltoid

Cutaneous nerve of shoulder

Posterior cutaneous branch of
radial n.

N. to long head of triceps

N. to triceps (lateral head)

N. to medial head of triceps

Posterior cutaneous nerve of forearm

N. to anconeus

N. to lateral fibres of brachialis

Olecranon

N. to brachio-radialis

Posterior interosseous nerve
(muscular)

N. to extensor carpi radialis longus

Radial nerve [ramus superficialis]

N. to extensor digitorum
[communis]

N. to extensor carpi radialis brevis

N. to extensor digiti minimi

N. to supinator

N. to extensor carpi ulnaris

N. to abductor pollicis longus

N. to extensor indicis

N. to extensor pollicis longus

N. to extensor pollicis brevis

Nerves to wrist joint and
intercarpal joints

PLATE 284.—ARTERIES OF UPPER LIMB
ANTERIOR ASPECT

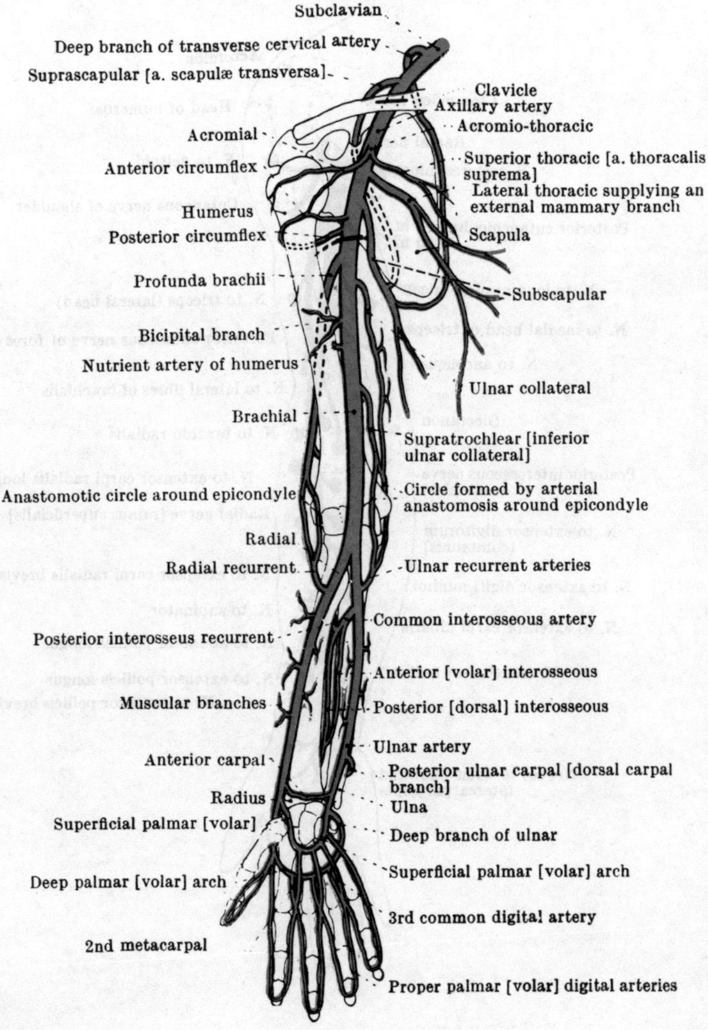

Subclavian

Deep branch of transverse cervical artery

Suprascapular [a. scapulæ transversa]

Clavicle
Axillary artery
Acromio-thoracic

Acromial

Anterior circumflex

Superior thoracic [a. thoracalis supremâ]
Lateral thoracic supplying an external mammary branch

Humerus
Posterior circumflex

Scapula

Profunda brachii

Subscapular

Bicipital branch
Nutrient artery of humerus

Ulnar collateral

Brachial

Supratrochlear [inferior ulnar collateral]

Anastomotic circle around epicondyle

Circle formed by arterial anastomosis around epicondyle

Radial
Radial recurrent

Ulnar recurrent arteries

Common interosseous artery

Posterior interosseus recurrent

Anterior [volar] interosseous

Muscular branches

Posterior [dorsal] interosseous

Ulnar artery

Anterior carpal

Posterior ulnar carpal [dorsal carpal branch]

Radius

Ulna

Superficial palmar [volar]

Deep branch of ulnar

Deep palmar [volar] arch

Superficial palmar [volar] arch

3rd common digital artery

2nd metacarpal

Proper palmar [volar] digital arteries

PLATE 285.—NERVES ON ANTERIOR [VOLAR] ASPECT OF HAND

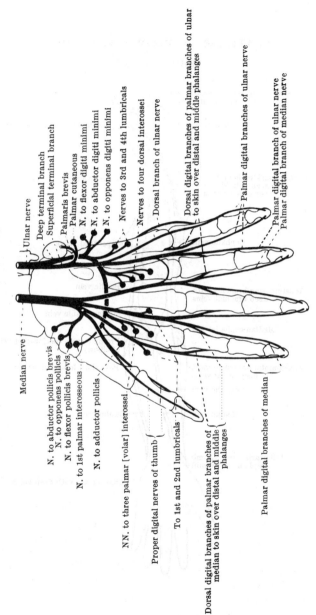

Median nerve

Ulnar nerve
Deep terminal branch
Superficial terminal branch
Palmaris brevis
Palmar cutaneous
N. to flexor digiti minimi
N. to abductor digiti minimi
N. to opponens digiti minimi

Nerves to 3rd and 4th lumbricals

Nerves to four dorsal interossei

Dorsal branch of ulnar nerve

Dorsal digital branches of palmar branches of ulnar
to skin over distal and middle phalanges

Palmar digital branches of ulnar nerve

Palmar digital branch of ulnar nerve
Palmar digital branch of median nerve

N. to abductor pollicis brevis
N. to opponens pollicis
N. to flexor pollicis brevis
N. to 1st palmar interosseous
N. to adductor pollicis

NN. to three palmar [volar] interossei

Proper digital nerves of thumb

To 1st and 2nd lumbricals

Dorsal digital branches of palmar branches of
median to skin over distal and middle
phalanges

Palmar digital branches of median

PLATE 286.—VEINS OF UPPER LIMB
ANTERIOR ASPECT

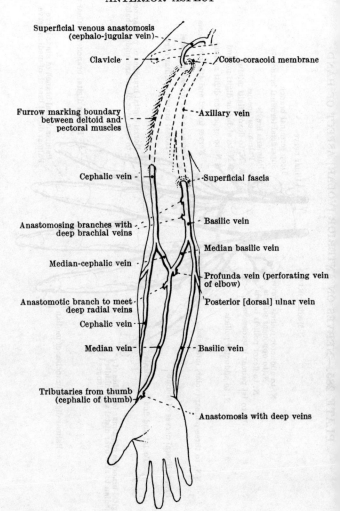

Superficial venous anastomosis (cephalo-jugular vein)

Clavicle

Costo-coracoid membrane

Furrow marking boundary between deltoid and pectoral muscles

Axillary vein

Cephalic vein

Superficial fascia

Anastomosing branches with deep brachial veins

Basilic vein

Median basilic vein

Median-cephalic vein

Profunda vein (perforating vein of elbow)

Anastomotic branch to meet deep radial veins

Posterior [dorsal] ulnar vein

Cephalic vein

Median vein

Basilic vein

Tributaries from thumb (cephalic of thumb)

Anastomosis with deep veins

PLATE 287.—VEINS OF UPPER LIMB
POSTERIOR OR DORSAL ASPECT

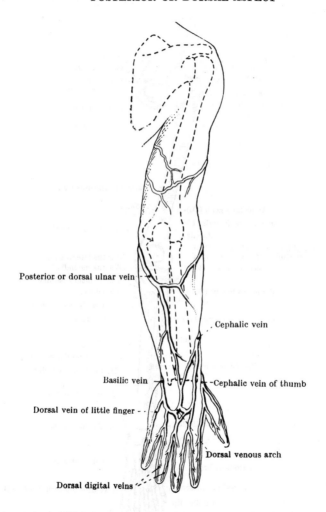

Posterior or dorsal ulnar vein

Cephalic vein

Basilic vein

Cephalic vein of thumb

Dorsal vein of little finger

Dorsal venous arch

Dorsal digital veins

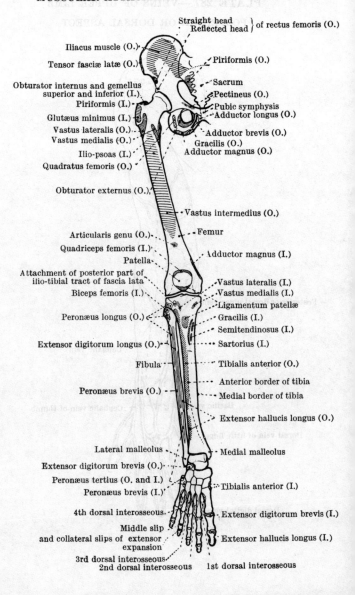

Straight head
Reflected head } of rectus femoris (O.)

Iliacus muscle (O.)

Tensor fasciæ latæ (O.)

Piriformis (O.)

Obturator internus and gemellus superior and inferior (I.)

Sacrum

Pectineus (O.)

Piriformis (I.)

Pubic symphysis

Glutæus minimus (I.)

Adductor longus (O.)

Vastus lateralis (O.)

Adductor brevis (O.)

Vastus medialis (O.)

Gracilis (O.)

Ilio-psoas (I.)

Adductor magnus (O.)

Quadratus femoris (O.)

Obturator externus (O.)

Vastus intermedius (O.)

Articularis genu (O.)

Femur

Quadriceps femoris (I.)

Adductor magnus (I.)

Patella

Attachment of posterior part of ilio-tibial tract of fascia lata

Vastus lateralis (I.)

Biceps femoris (I.)

Vastus medialis (I.)

Ligamentum patellæ

Peronæus longus (O.)

Gracilis (I.)

Semitendinosus (I.)

Extensor digitorum longus (O.)

Sartorius (I.)

Fibula

Tibialis anterior (O.)

Anterior border of tibia

Peronæus brevis (O.)

Medial border of tibia

Extensor hallucis longus (O.)

Lateral malleolus

Medial malleolus

Extensor digitorum brevis (O.)

Peronæus tertius (O. and I.)

Peronæus brevis (I.)

Tibialis anterior (I.)

4th dorsal interosseous

Extensor digitorum brevis (I.)

Middle slip and collateral slips of extensor expansion

Extensor hallucis longus (I.)

3rd dorsal interosseous

2nd dorsal interosseous

1st dorsal interosseous

Glutæus medius (O.)

Glutæus minimus (O.)

Reflected tendon of rectus femoris (O.)

Glutæus maximus (O.)

Gemellus superior (O.)

Gemellus inferior (O.)

Obturator internus (O.)

Semimembranosus (O.)

Biceps femoris (long head) (O.)

Obturator externus (I.)

Glutæus medius (I.)

Quadratus femoris (I.)

Ilio-psoas (I.)

Semitendinosus (O.)

Pectineus (I.)

Adductor brevis (I.)

Glutæus maximus (I.)

Adductor longus (I.)

Vastus intermedius (O.)

Vastus medialis (O.)

Vastus lateralis (O.)

Biceps femoris (short head) (O.)

Adductor magnus (I.)

Plantaris (O.)

Gastrocnemius (medial head) (O.)

Gastrocnemius (lateral head) (O.)

Popliteus (O.)

Femur : medial condyle

Membranous insertion of semimembranosus entering into formation of oblique ligament

Tendinous insertion of semimembranosus

Soleus (O.)

Tibialis posterior (O.)

Popliteus (I.)

Flexor hallucis longus (O.)

Flexor digitorum longus (O.)

Tibia

Peronæus brevis (O.)

Fibula

Attachment of tendo calcaneus and of tendon of plantaris

Abductor digiti minimi (O.)

Accessory slip of flexor digitorum longus (I.)

Flexor digitorum brevis (O.)

Abductor hallucis (O.)

Flexor digiti minimi brevis (O.)

Tibialis posterior (I.)

Tibialis anterior (I.)

Adductor hallucis (O.)

Peronæus longus (I.)

Flexor digitorum brevis and abductor digiti minimi (I.)

Abductor hallucis (I.)

Flexor hallucis brevis (O. and I.)

Adductor hallucis (I.)

3rd plantar interosseous

Flexor hallucis longus (I.)

2nd plantar interosseous

Flexor digitorum brevis (I.)

1st plantar interosseous

Flexor digitorum longus (I.)

19

PLATE 290.—MUSCLES OF THE LOWER LIMB

ANTERIOR ASPECT

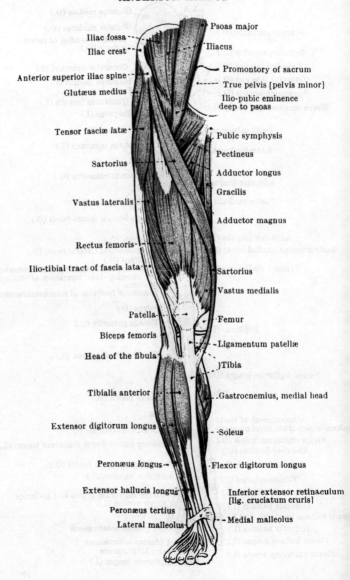

Iliac fossa

Iliac crest

Anterior superior iliac spine

Glutæus medius

Tensor fasciæ latæ

Sartorius

Vastus lateralis

Rectus femoris

Ilio-tibial tract of fascia lata

Patella

Biceps femoris

Head of the fibula

Tibialis anterior

Extensor digitorum longus

Peronæus longus

Extensor hallucis longus

Peronæus tertius

Lateral malleolus

Psoas major

Iliacus

Promontory of sacrum

True pelvis [pelvis minor]

Ilio-pubic eminence deep to psoas

Pubic symphysis

Pectineus

Adductor longus

Gracilis

Adductor magnus

Sartorius

Vastus medialis

Femur

Ligamentum patellæ

Tibia

Gastrocnemius, medial head

Soleus

Flexor digitorum longus

Inferior extensor retinaculum [lig. cruciatum cruris]

Medial malleolus

PLATE 291.—MUSCLES OF THE LOWER LIMB
POSTERIOR ASPECT

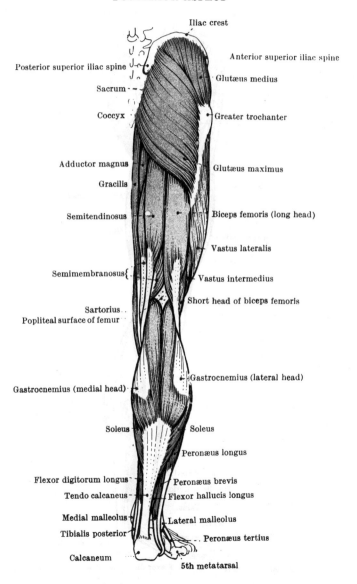

Iliac crest

Anterior superior iliac spine

Posterior superior iliac spine

Glutæus medius

Sacrum

Coccyx

Greater trochanter

Adductor magnus

Glutæus maximus

Gracilis

Semitendinosus

Biceps femoris (long head)

Vastus lateralis

Vastus intermedius

Semimembranosus{

Short head of biceps femoris

Sartorius
Popliteal surface of femur

Gastrocnemius (lateral head)

Gastrocnemius (medial head)

Soleus

Soleus

Peronæus longus

Flexor digitorum longus

Peronæus brevis

Tendo calcaneus

Flexor hallucis longus

Medial malleolus

Lateral malleolus

Tibialis posterior

Peronæus tertius

Calcaneum

5th metatarsal

PLATE 292.—MUSCLES OF THE LOWER LIMB
MEDIAL ASPECT

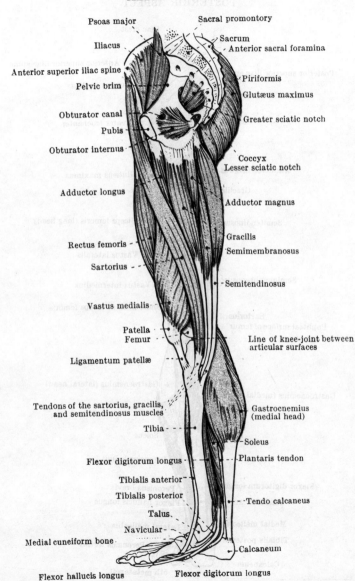

Psoas major

Iliacus

Anterior superior iliac spine

Pelvic brim

Obturator canal

Pubis

Obturator internus

Adductor longus

Rectus femoris

Sartorius

Vastus medialis

Patella
Femur

Ligamentum patellæ

Tendons of the sartorius, gracilis,
and semitendinosus muscles

Tibia

Flexor digitorum longus

Tibialis anterior

Tibialis posterior

Talus

Navicular

Medial cuneiform bone

Flexor hallucis longus

Sacral promontory

Sacrum
Anterior sacral foramina

Piriformis

Glutæus maximus

Greater sciatic notch

Coccyx
Lesser sciatic notch

Adductor magnus

Gracilis
Semimembranosus

Semitendinosus

Line of knee-joint between
articular surfaces

Gastrocnemius
(medial head)

Soleus

Plantaris tendon

Tendo calcaneus

Calcaneum

Flexor digitorum longus

PLATE 293.—MUSCLES OF THE LOWER LIMB
LATERAL ASPECT

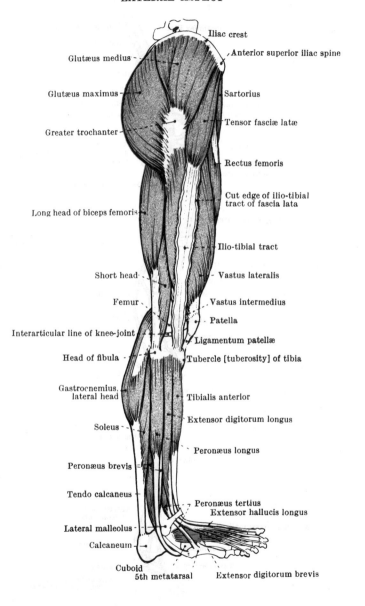

Iliac crest

Anterior superior iliac spine

Glutæus medius

Glutæus maximus

Sartorius

Greater trochanter

Tensor fasciæ latæ

Rectus femoris

Cut edge of ilio-tibial
tract of fascia lata

Long head of biceps femoris

Ilio-tibial tract

Short head

Vastus lateralis

Femur

Vastus intermedius

Patella

Interarticular line of knee-joint

Ligamentum patellæ

Head of fibula

Tubercle [tuberosity] of tibia

Gastrocnemius,
lateral head

Tibialis anterior

Extensor digitorum longus

Soleus

Peronæus longus

Peronæus brevis

Tendo calcaneus

Peronæus tertius
Extensor hallucis longus

Lateral malleolus

Calcaneum

Cuboid
5th metatarsal

Extensor digitorum brevis

PLATE 294.—ARTERIES OF THE LOWER LIMB
ANTERIOR ASPECT

Anastomotic branch to deep circumflex iliac

Common iliac artery

Superficial epigastric

Superficial circumflex iliac art.

Art. to quadriceps

Internal iliac [hypogastric]

External iliac

Superficial external pudendal

Medial circumflex artery

Obturator artery

Pubic symphysis

Anastomosis

Lateral circumflex artery

Anastomosis with internal pudendal

Profunda artery

Deep external pudendal

Perforating arteries

Femoral artery

Femur

Descending genicular [a. genu suprema]

Femoral artery leaving subsartorial canal [through opening in adductor magnus]

Anastomosis in front of knee

Superior medial genicular artery

Superior lateral genicular artery

Patella

Anastomosis

Anastomosis

Inferior lateral genicular

Inferior medial genicular artery

Anastomosis

Anterior tibial recurrent artery

Tibia

Anterior tibial artery

Muscular branches

Fibula

Anterior medial malleolar art.

Anterior lateral malleolar artery

Anastomosis

Anastomosis

Tarsal artery

Dorsalis pedis artery

Arcuate artery giving off dorsal metatarsal arteries

PLATE 295.—ARTERIES OF THE LOWER LIMB
POSTERIOR ASPECT

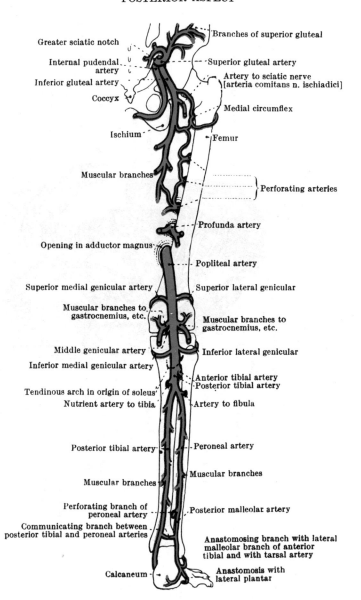

Branches of superior gluteal

Greater sciatic notch

Internal pudendal artery

Superior gluteal artery

Inferior gluteal artery

Artery to sciatic nerve [arteria comitans n. ischiadici]

Coccyx

Medial circumflex

Ischium

Femur

Muscular branches

Perforating arteries

Profunda artery

Opening in adductor magnus

Popliteal artery

Superior medial genicular artery

Superior lateral genicular

Muscular branches to gastrocnemius, etc.

Muscular branches to gastrocnemius, etc.

Middle genicular artery

Inferior lateral genicular

Inferior medial genicular artery

Anterior tibial artery
Posterior tibial artery

Tendinous arch in origin of soleus

Nutrient artery to tibia

Artery to fibula

Posterior tibial artery

Peroneal artery

Muscular branches

Muscular branches

Perforating branch of peroneal artery

Posterior malleolar artery

Communicating branch between posterior tibial and peroneal arteries

Anastomosing branch with lateral malleolar branch of anterior tibial and with tarsal artery

Calcaneum

Anastomosis with lateral plantar

PLATE 296.—GLUTEAL REGION

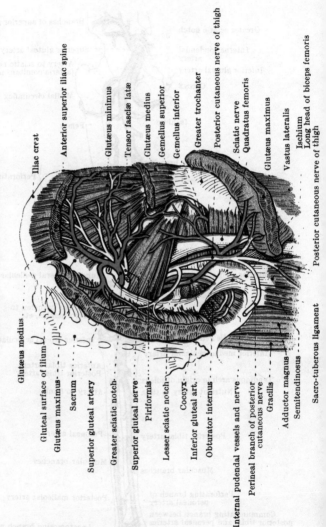

Iliac crest
Anterior superior iliac spine
Gluteus minimus
Tensor fasciae latae
Gluteus medius
Gemellus superior
Gemellus inferior
Greater trochanter
Posterior cutaneous nerve of thigh
Sciatic nerve
Quadratus femoris
Gluteus maximus
Vastus lateralis
Ischium
Long head of biceps femoris

Gluteus medius
Gluteal surface of ilium
Gluteus maximus
Sacrum
Superior gluteal artery
Greater sciatic notch
Superior gluteal nerve
Piriformis
Lesser sciatic notch
Coccyx
Inferior gluteal art.
Obturator internus
Internal pudendal vessels and nerve
Perineal branch of posterior cutaneous nerve
Gracilis
Adductor magnus
Semitendinosus
Sacro-tuberous ligament
Posterior cutaneous nerve of thigh

PLATE 297.—QUADRICEPS EXTENSOR

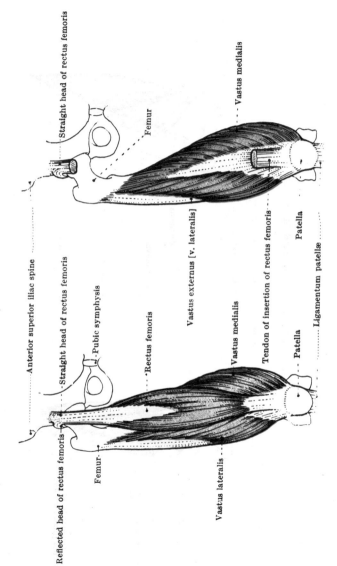

Anterior superior iliac spine

Straight head of rectus femoris

Straight head of rectus femoris

Pubic symphysis

Femur

Rectus femoris

Vastus externus [v. lateralis]

Vastus medialis

Vastus medialis

Tendon of insertion of rectus femoris

Reflected head of rectus femoris

Patella

Patella

Femur

Ligamentum patellæ

Vastus lateralis

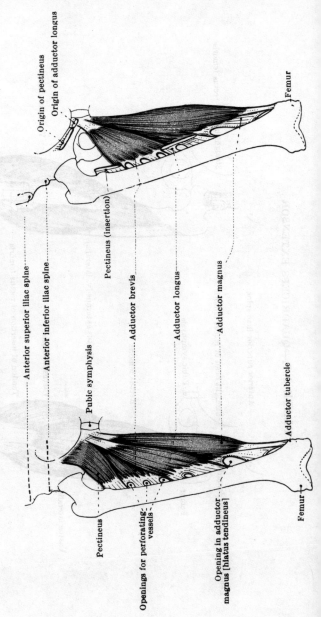

PLATE 298.—ADDUCTOR MUSCLES

Anterior superior iliac spine
Anterior inferior iliac spine
Origin of pectineus
Origin of adductor longus
Pubic symphysis
Pectineus (insertion)
Adductor brevis
Adductor longus
Adductor magnus
Femur
Adductor tubercle
Pectineus
Openings for perforating vessels
Opening in adductor magnus [hiatus tendineus]
Femur

PLATE 299.—MUSCLES OF THE LOWER LIMB
POSTERIOR ASPECT

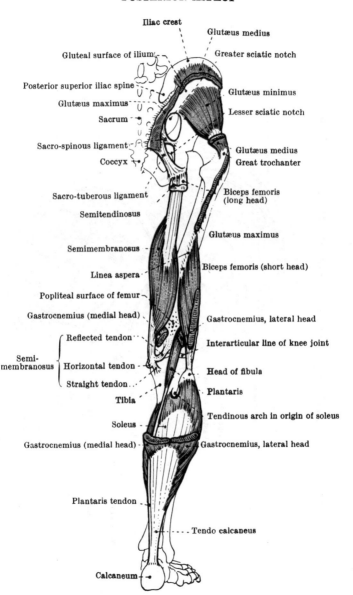

Iliac crest

Glutæus medius

Gluteal surface of ilium

Greater sciatic notch

Posterior superior iliac spine

Glutæus minimus

Glutæus maximus

Lesser sciatic notch

Sacrum

Sacro-spinous ligament

Glutæus medius

Coccyx

Great trochanter

Sacro-tuberous ligament

Biceps femoris (long head)

Semitendinosus

Glutæus maximus

Semimembranosus

Linea aspera

Biceps femoris (short head)

Popliteal surface of femur

Gastrocnemius (medial head)

Gastrocnemius, lateral head

Reflected tendon

Interarticular line of knee joint

Semi-membranosus { Horizontal tendon

Head of fibula

Straight tendon

Plantaris

Tibia

Tendinous arch in origin of soleus

Soleus

Gastrocnemius (medial head)

Gastrocnemius, lateral head

Plantaris tendon

Tendo calcaneus

Calcaneum

PLATE 300.—SECTION THROUGH MIDDLE OF THIGH

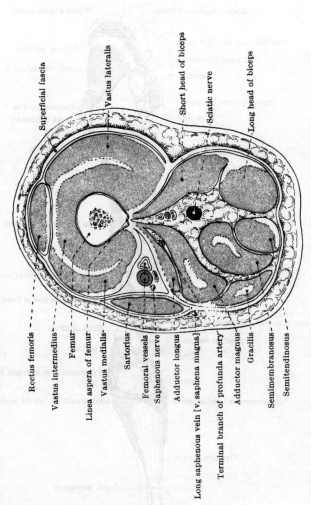

Rectus femoris
Vastus intermedius
Femur
Linea aspera of femur
Vastus medialis
Sartorius
Femoral vessels
Saphenous nerve
Long saphenous vein [v. saphena magna]
Terminal branch of profunda artery
Adductor magnus
Gracilis
Semimembranosus
Semitendinosus

Superficial fascia
Vastus lateralis
Short head of biceps
Sciatic nerve
Long head of biceps
Adductor longus

PLATE 301.—SECTION THROUGH LEG—UPPER PART

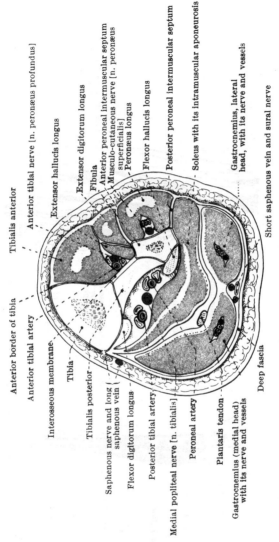

Anterior border of tibia

Tibialis anterior

Anterior tibial nerve [n. peroneus profundus]

Extensor hallucis longus

Extensor digitorum longus

Fibula

Anterior peroneal intermuscular septum

Musculo-cutaneous nerve [n. peroneus superficialis]

Peronaeus longus

Flexor hallucis longus

Posterior peroneal intermuscular septum

Soleus with its intramuscular aponeurosis

Gastrocnemius, lateral head, with its nerve and vessels

Short saphenous vein and sural nerve

Anterior tibial artery

Interosseous membrane

Tibia

Tibialis posterior

Saphenous nerve and long saphenous vein

Flexor digitorum longus

Posterior tibial artery

Medial popliteal nerve [n. tibialis]

Peroneal artery

Plantaris tendon

Gastrocnemius (medial head) with its nerve and vessels

Deep fascia

PLATE 302.—MUSCLES OF THE LEG AND FOOT—ANTERIOR ASPECT

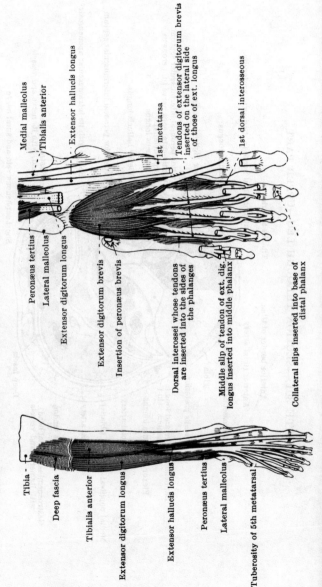

Tibia

Deep fascia

Tibialis anterior

Extensor digitorum longus

Extensor hallucis longus

Peronaeus tertius

Lateral malleolus

Tuberosity of 5th metatarsal

Medial malleolus
Tibialis anterior

Extensor hallucis longus

Peronaeus tertius
Lateral malleolus

Extensor digitorum longus

1st metatarsal

Tendons of extensor digitorum brevis
inserted on the lateral side
of those of ext. longus

Extensor digitorum brevis

Insertion of peronaeus brevis

1st dorsal interosseous

Dorsal interossei whose tendons
are inserted into the sides of
the phalanges

Middle slip of tendon of ext. dig.
longus inserted into middle phalanx

Collateral slips inserted into base of
distal phalanx

PLATE 303.—MUSCLES OF THE LEG AND FOOT—POSTERIOR ASPECT

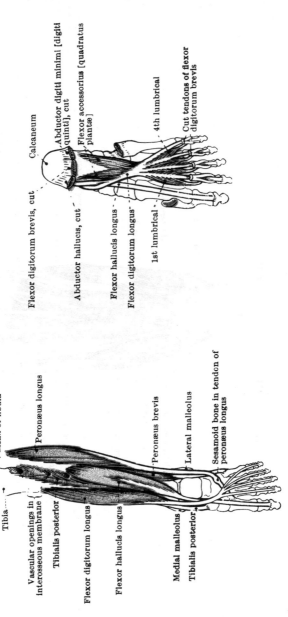

PLATE 304.—MUSCLES OF SOLE OF FOOT

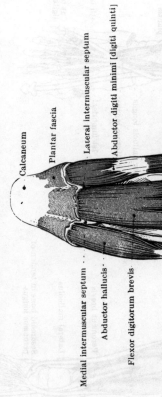

Calcaneum

Plantar fascia

Lateral intermuscular septum

Abductor digiti minimi [digiti quinti]

Tendons of flexor digitorum longus

4th lumbrical

Tendons (perforated) of flexor digitorum brevis

Tendons (perforating) of flexor digitorum longus

Medial intermuscular septum

Abductor hallucis

Flexor digitorum brevis

Flexor hallucis brevis {medial portion / lateral portion

Prominence of sesamoid bones

1st lumbrical

Tendon of flexor hallucis longus

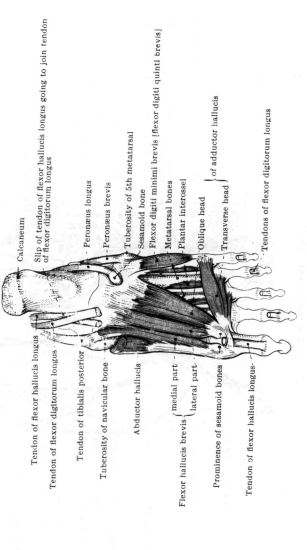

PLATE 305 — MUSCLES OF SOLE OF FOOT [DEEP DISSECTION]

Calcaneum

Slip of tendon of flexor hallucis longus going to join tendon of flexor digitorum longus

Peronaeus longus

Peronaeus brevis

Tuberosity of 5th metatarsal

Sesamoid bone

Flexor digiti minimi brevis [flexor digiti quinti brevis]

Metatarsal bones

Plantar interossei

Oblique head ⎫
Transverse head ⎭ of adductor hallucis

Tendons of flexor digitorum longus

Tendon of flexor hallucis longus

Tendon of flexor digitorum longus

Tendon of tibialis posterior

Tuberosity of navicular bone

Abductor hallucis

Flexor hallucis brevis ⎰medial part
⎱lateral part

Prominence of sesamoid bones

Tendon of flexor hallucis longus

PLATE 306.—INGUINAL REGION

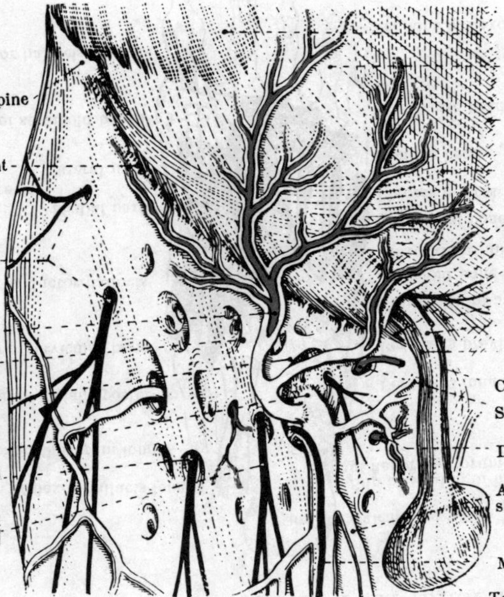

Obliquus externus abdominis

Its aponeurosis

Linea alba

Rectus abdominis (seen through sheath)

Cutaneous branch of ilio-inguinal nerve
Genital branch of genito-femoral [n. spermaticus externus]
Inferior crus of superficial inguinal ring

Superior crus

External spermatic fascia

Cremaster muscle

Superficial external pudendal artery

Deep external pudendal artery

Anastomosis between long and short saphenous veins

Medial cutaneous nerve

Testis

Anterior superior iliac spine

Inguinal ligament

Branches of lateral cutaneous nerve

Superficial epigastric artery

Cribriform fascia

Falciform margin of saphenous opening (fossa ovalis)

Long saphenous vein [v. saphena magna]

Intermediate cutaneous nerve of femoral

Femoral branch of genito-femoral nerve [n. lumbo-inguinalis]

PLATE 307.—INGUINAL REGION AND FEMORAL TRIANGLE

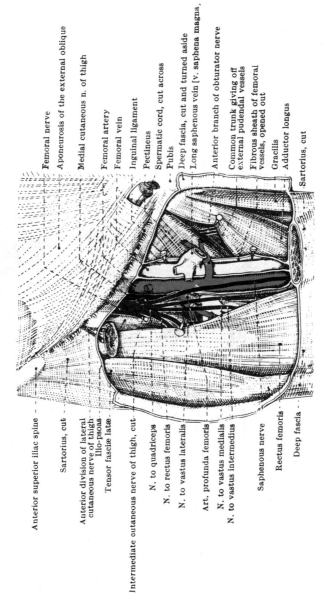

Anterior superior iliac spine

Sartorius, cut

Anterior division of lateral
cutaneous nerve of thigh

Ilio-psoas

Tensor fasciae latae

Intermediate cutaneous nerve of thigh, cut

N. to quadriceps

N. to rectus femoris

N. to vastus lateralis

Art. profunda femoris

N. to vastus medialis

N. to vastus intermedius

Saphenous nerve

Rectus femoris

Deep fascia

Femoral nerve

Aponeurosis of the external oblique

Medial cutaneous n. of thigh

Femoral artery

Femoral vein

Inguinal ligament

Pectineus

Spermatic cord, cut across

Pubis

Deep fascia, cut and turned aside

Long saphenous vein [v. saphena magna,

Anterior branch of obturator nerve

Common trunk giving off
external pudendal vessels

Fibrous sheath of femoral
vessels, opened out

Gracilis

Adductor longus

Sartorius, cut

PLATE 308.—FRONT OF THIGH

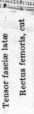

Tensor fasciae latae

Rectus femoris, cut

Vessels and nerve to the quadriceps

Ilio-tibial tract

Vastus lateralis

Vastus intermedius

Rectus femoris, cut

Tendon of quadriceps

Sartorius, cut

Gracilis

Adductor longus

Adductor magnus

Femoral vein

Femoral artery

Roof of subsartorial [adductor] canal, laid open

Fibrous septum between femoral artery and vein

Branch of saphenous nerve to subsartorial plexus

Subsartorial canal [c. adductorius]

Descending genicular art. [a. genu suprema]

Saphenous nerve

Vastus medialis

Sartorius, cut

PLATE 309 — BACK OF THIGH

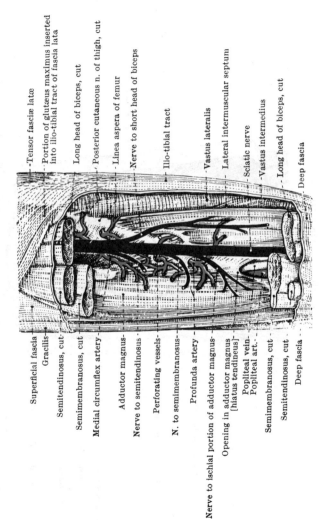

Tensor fasciae latae

Portion of gluteus maximus inserted into ilio-tibial tract of fascia lata

Long head of biceps, cut

Posterior cutaneous n. of thigh, cut

Linea aspera of femur

Nerve to short head of biceps

Ilio-tibial tract

Vastus lateralis

Lateral intermuscular septum

Sciatic nerve

Vastus intermedius

Long head of biceps, cut

Deep fascia

Superficial fascia

Gracilis

Semitendinosus, cut

Semimembranosus, cut

Medial circumflex artery

Adductor magnus

Nerve to semitendinosus

Perforating vessels

N. to semimembranosus

Profunda artery

Nerve to ischial portion of adductor magnus

Opening in adductor magnus [hiatus tendineus]

Popliteal vein
Popliteal art.

Semimembranosus, cut

Semitendinosus, cut

Deep fascia

PLATE 310.—FRONT OF KNEE

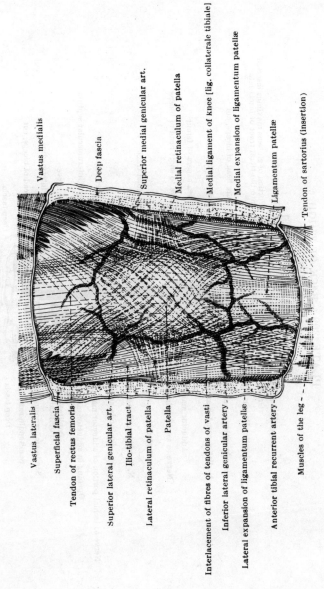

Vastus medialis

Deep fascia

Superior medial genicular art.

Medial retinaculum of patella

Medial ligament of knee [lig. collaterale tibiale]

Medial expansion of ligamentum patellæ

Ligamentum patellæ

Tendon of sartorius (insertion)

Vastus lateralis

Superficial fascia

Tendon of rectus femoris

Superior lateral genicular art.

Ilio-tibial tract

Lateral retinaculum of patella

Patella

Interlacement of fibres of tendons of vasti

Inferior lateral genicular artery

Lateral expansion of ligamentum patellæ

Anterior tibial recurrent artery

Muscles of the leg

PLATE 311.—BACK OF KNEE

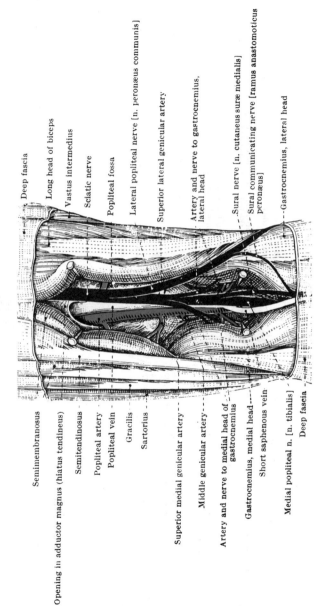

Semimembranosus

Opening in adductor magnus (hiatus tendineus)

Semitendinosus

Popliteal artery

Popliteal vein

Gracilis

Sartorius

Superior medial genicular artery

Middle genicular artery

Artery and nerve to medial head of gastrocnemius

Gastrocnemius, medial head

Short saphenous vein

Medial popliteal n. [n. tibialis]

Deep fascia

Deep fascia

Long head of biceps

Vastus intermedius

Sciatic nerve

Popliteal fossa

Lateral popliteal nerve [n. peronaeus communis]

Superior lateral genicular artery

Artery and nerve to gastrocnemius, lateral head

Sural nerve [n. cutaneus surae medialis]

Sural communicating nerve [ramus anastomoticus peronaeus]

Gastrocnemius, lateral head

PLATE 312.—FRONT OF LEG

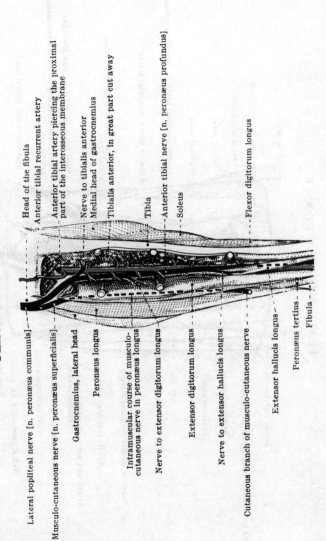

Lateral popliteal nerve [n. peronæus communis]

Musculo-cutaneous nerve [n. peronæus superficialis]

Gastrocnemius, lateral head

Peronæus longus

Intramuscular course of musculo-
cutaneous nerve in peronæus longus

Nerve to extensor digitorum longus

Extensor digitorum longus

Nerve to extensor hallucis longus

Cutaneous branch of musculo-cutaneous nerve

Extensor hallucis longus

Peronæus tertius

Fibula

Head of the fibula

Anterior tibial recurrent artery

Anterior tibial artery piercing the proximal
part of the interosseous membrane

Nerve to tibialis anterior

Medial head of gastrocnemius

Tibialis anterior, in great part cut away

Tibia

Anterior tibial nerve [n. peronæus profundus]

Soleus

Flexor digitorum longus

PLATE 313.—BACK OF LEG

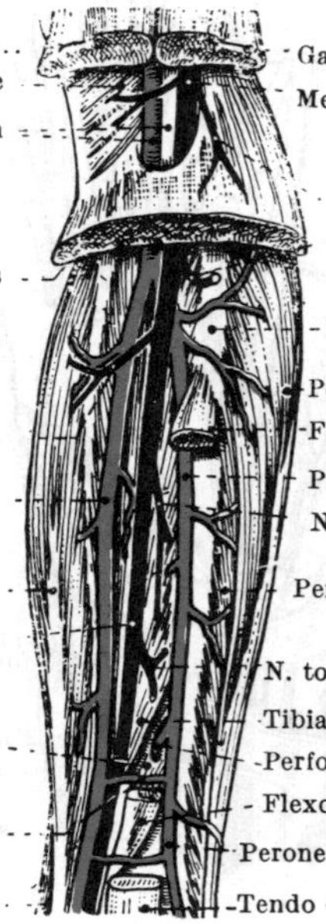

Gastrocnemius, medial head
Popliteus muscle with its nerve
Popliteal artery and vein

Gastrocnemius, lateral head
Medial popliteal nerve [n. tibialis]

Upper and lower branches to soleus

Fibrous arch (arcus tendineus) of soleus

Fibula
Peronæus longus
Flexor hallucis longus
Peroneal artery
N. to tibialis posterior

Peronæus brevis

N. to flexor hallucis longus

Tibialis posterior
Perforating branch of peroneal artery
Flexor hallucis longus
Peroneal artery terminating as lateral calcanean branches
Tendo calcaneus

N. to flexor digitorum longus
Posterior tibial artery

Flexor digitorum longus
Posterior tibial nerve

Interosseous membrane

Arterial anastomosis

Tibialis posterior

PLATE 314.—DORSUM OF FOOT

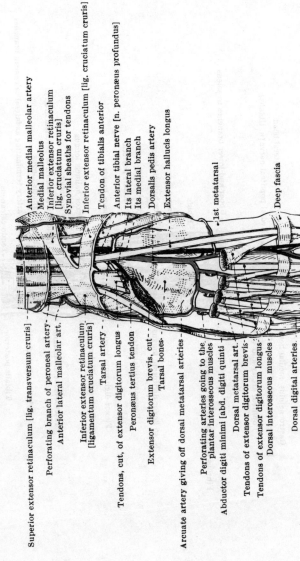

Superior extensor retinaculum [lig. transversum cruris]

Perforating branch of peroneal artery

Anterior lateral malleolar art.

Inferior extensor retinaculum [ligamentum cruciatum cruris]

Tarsal artery

Tendons, cut, of extensor digitorum longus

Peronæus tertius tendon

Extensor digitorum brevis, cut

Tarsal bones

Arcuate artery giving off dorsal metatarsal arteries

Perforating arteries going to the plantar interosseous muscles

Abductor digiti minimi [abd. digiti quinti]

Dorsal metatarsal art.

Tendons of extensor digitorum brevis

Tendons of extensor digitorum longus

Dorsal interosseous muscles

Dorsal digital arteries.

Anterior medial malleolar artery

Medial malleolus

Inferior extensor retinaculum [lig. cruciatum cruris]

Synovial sheaths for tendons

Inferior extensor retinaculum [lig. cruciatum cruris]

Tendon of tibialis anterior

Anterior tibial nerve [n. peronæus profundus]

Its lateral branch

Its medial branch

Dorsalis pedis artery

Extensor hallucis longus

1st metatarsal

Deep fascia

PLATE 315.—SOLE OF FOOT

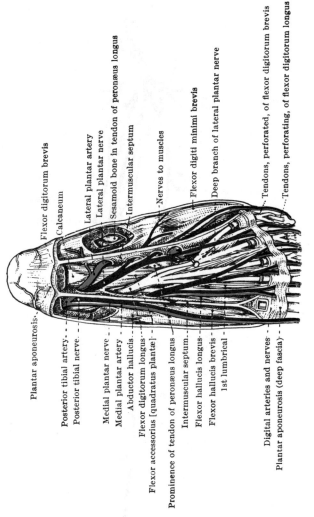

Plantar aponeurosis.

Flexor digitorum brevis

Calcaneum

Lateral plantar artery

Lateral plantar nerve

Sesamoid bone in tendon of peronaeus longus

Intermuscular septum

Nerves to muscles

Flexor digiti minimi brevis

Deep branch of lateral plantar nerve

Tendons, perforated, of flexor digitorum brevis

Tendons, perforating, of flexor digitorum longus

Posterior tibial artery.

Posterior tibial nerve.

Medial plantar nerve

Medial plantar artery

Abductor hallucis.

Flexor digitorum longus

Flexor accessorius [quadratus plantae]

Prominence of tendon of peronaeus longus

Intermuscular septum.

Flexor hallucis longus

Flexor hallucis brevis

1st lumbrical

Digital arteries and nerves

Plantar aponeurosis (deep fascia)

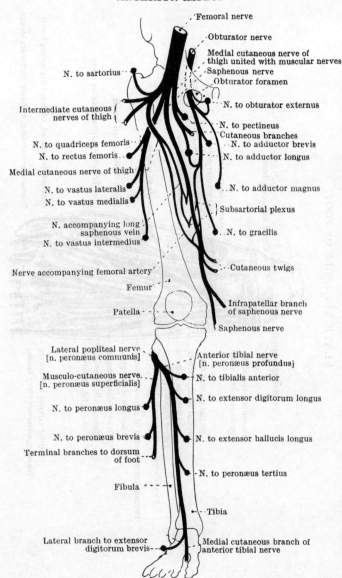

PLATE 316.—NERVES OF LOWER LIMB
ANTERIOR ASPECT

Femoral nerve

Obturator nerve

Medial cutaneous nerve of thigh united with muscular nerves

Saphenous nerve

Obturator foramen

N. to sartorius

N. to obturator externus

Intermediate cutaneous nerves of thigh

N. to pectineus

Cutaneous branches

N. to adductor brevis

N. to quadriceps femoris

N. to adductor longus

N. to rectus femoris

Medial cutaneous nerve of thigh

N. to vastus lateralis

N. to adductor magnus

N. to vastus medialis

Subsartorial plexus

N. accompanying long saphenous vein

N. to gracilis

N. to vastus intermedius

Cutaneous twigs

Nerve accompanying femoral artery

Femur

Infrapatellar branch of saphenous nerve

Patella

Saphenous nerve

Lateral popliteal nerve [n. peronæus communis]

Anterior tibial nerve [n. peronæus profundus]

Musculo-cutaneous nerve [n. peronæus superficialis]

N. to tibialis anterior

N. to extensor digitorum longus

N. to peronæus longus

N. to extensor hallucis longus

N. to peronæus brevis

Terminal branches to dorsum of foot

N. to peronæus tertius

Fibula

Tibia

Lateral branch to extensor digitorum brevis

Medial cutaneous branch of anterior tibial nerve

PLATE 317.—NERVES OF LOWER LIMB
POSTERIOR ASPECT

N. to glutæus medius

Superior gluteal nerve

N. to glutæus minimus

N. to m. tensor fasciæ latæ

Greater sciatic notch

Sacral plexus

N. to piriformis

Inferior gluteal nerve to glutæus maximus

N. to gemellus superior

N. to gemellus inferior

Perineal nerve

Sciatic nerve

Posterior cutaneous nerve of thigh

N. to quadratus femoris

Femur

N. to long head of biceps femoris

N. to short head of biceps femoris

N. to semitendinosus

N. to semimembranosus

N. to adductor magnus

Lateral popliteal nerve [n. peronæus communis]

Medial popliteal nerve [n. tibialis]

Lateral cutaneous nerve of calf

N. to popliteus

Head of fibula

NN. to two heads of gastrocnemius

N. to plantaris

Sural nerve [ramus communicans tibialis

N. to soleus

Sural communicating nerve [n. peronæus anastomoticus]

Tendinous arch of soleus

N. to tibialis posterior

Sural nerve

N. to flexor hallucis longus

N. to flexor digitorum longus

Posterior tibial nerve

Tibia

Medial calcanean nerve

PLATE 318.—VEINS OF LOWER LIMB
ANTERIOR ASPECT

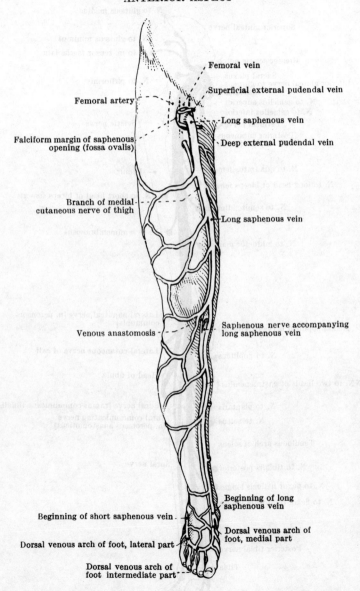

Femoral artery

Falciform margin of saphenous opening (fossa ovalis)

Branch of medial cutaneous nerve of thigh

Venous anastomosis

Beginning of short saphenous vein

Dorsal venous arch of foot, lateral part

Dorsal venous arch of foot intermediate part

Femoral vein

Superficial external pudendal vein

Long saphenous vein

Deep external pudendal vein

Long saphenous vein

Saphenous nerve accompanying long saphenous vein

Beginning of long saphenous vein

Dorsal venous arch of foot, medial part

PLATE 319.—VEINS OF LOWER LIMB
POSTERIOR ASPECT

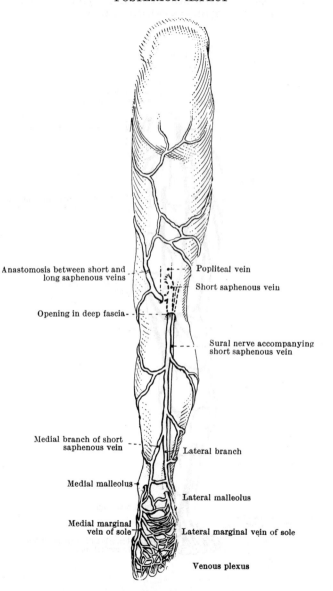

Anastomosis between short and long saphenous veins

Popliteal vein

Short saphenous vein

Opening in deep fascia

Sural nerve accompanying short saphenous vein

Medial branch of short saphenous vein

Lateral branch

Medial malleolus

Lateral malleolus

Medial marginal vein of sole

Lateral marginal vein of sole

Venous plexus

PLATE 320.—SUPERFICIAL (CUTANEOUS) NERVES OF
LOWER LIMB—ANTERIOR ASPECT

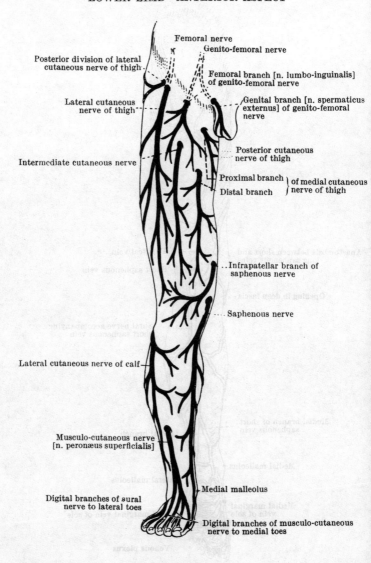

Femoral nerve

Genito-femoral nerve

Posterior division of lateral
cutaneous nerve of thigh

Femoral branch [n. lumbo-inguinalis]
of genito-femoral nerve

Lateral cutaneous
nerve of thigh

Genital branch [n. spermaticus
externus] of genito-femoral
nerve

Posterior cutaneous
nerve of thigh

Intermediate cutaneous nerve

Proximal branch ⎫ of medial cutaneous
Distal branch ⎭ nerve of thigh

Infrapatellar branch of
saphenous nerve

Saphenous nerve

Lateral cutaneous nerve of calf

Musculo-cutaneous nerve
[n. peronæus superficialis]

Medial malleolus

Digital branches of sural
nerve to lateral toes

Digital branches of musculo-cutaneous
nerve to medial toes

PLATE 321.—SUPERFICIAL (CUTANEOUS) NERVES
OF LOWER LIMB—POSTERIOR ASPECT

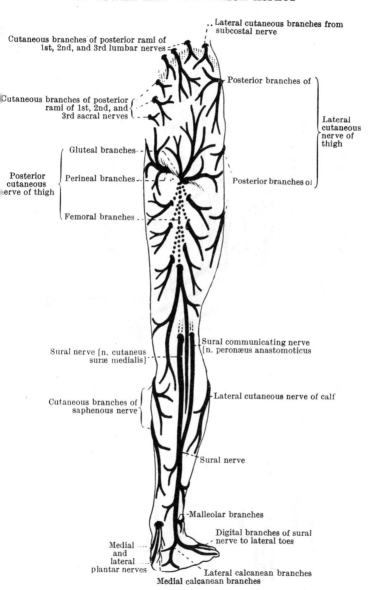

Lateral cutaneous branches from subcostal nerve

Cutaneous branches of posterior rami of 1st, 2nd, and 3rd lumbar nerves

Posterior branches of

Cutaneous branches of posterior rami of 1st, 2nd, and 3rd sacral nerves

Lateral cutaneous nerve of thigh

Gluteal branches

Posterior cutaneous nerve of thigh

Perineal branches

Posterior branches of

Femoral branches

Sural communicating nerve [n. peronæus anastomoticus]

Sural nerve [n. cutaneus suræ medialis]

Lateral cutaneous nerve of calf

Cutaneous branches of saphenous nerve

Sural nerve

Malleolar branches

Digital branches of sural nerve to lateral toes

Medial and lateral plantar nerves

Lateral calcanean branches

Medial calcanean branches

21

PLATE 322.—LYMPHATICS OF NASAL CAVITIES

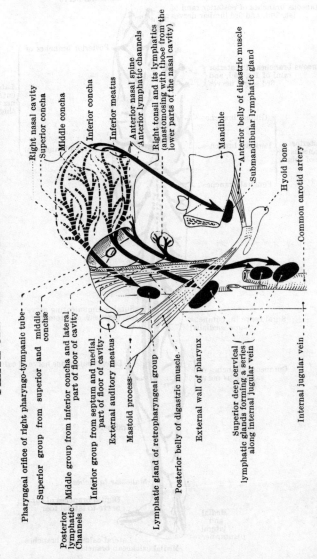

Pharyngeal orifice of right pharyngo-tympanic tube

Superior group from superior and middle concha — Posterior lymphatic Channels

Middle group from inferior concha and lateral part of floor of cavity

Inferior group from septum and medial part of floor of cavity

External auditory meatus

Mastoid process

Lymphatic gland of retropharyngeal group

Posterior belly of digastric muscle

External wall of pharynx

Superior deep cervical lymphatic glands forming a series along internal jugular vein

Internal jugular vein

Right nasal cavity
Superior concha
Middle concha
Inferior concha
Inferior meatus
Anterior nasal spine
Anterior lymphatic channels
Right tonsil and its lymphatics (anastomosing with those from the lower parts of the nasal cavity)
Mandible
Anterior belly of digastric muscle
Submandibular lymphatic gland
Hyoid bone
Common carotid artery

PLATE 323.—LYMPHATICS OF TONGUE

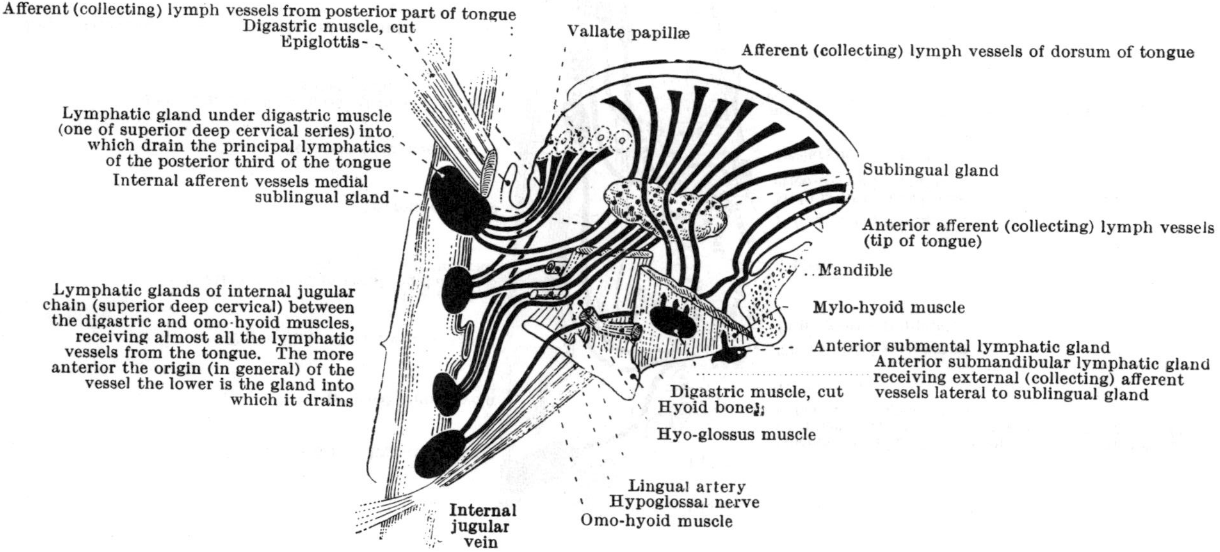

Afferent (collecting) lymph vessels from posterior part of tongue

Digastric muscle, cut

Epiglottis

Vallate papillae

Afferent (collecting) lymph vessels of dorsum of tongue

Sublingual gland

Anterior afferent (collecting) lymph vessels

Mandible

Anterior afferent (collecting) lymph vessels (tip of tongue)

Mylo-hyoid muscle

Anterior submental lymphatic gland

Anterior submandibular lymphatic gland receiving external (collecting) afferent vessels lateral to sublingual gland

Digastric muscle, cut

Hyoid bone‡;

Hyo-glossus muscle

Lingual artery

Hypoglossal nerve

Omo-hyoid muscle

Lymphatic gland under digastric muscle (one of superior deep cervical series) into which drain the principal lymphatics of the posterior third of the tongue

Internal afferent vessels medial sublingual gland

Internal jugular vein

Lymphatic glands of internal jugular chain (superior deep cervical) between the digastric and omo-hyoid muscles, receiving almost all the lymphatic vessels from the tongue. The more anterior the origin (in general) of the vessel the lower is the gland into which it drains

PLATE 324.—LYMPHATICS OF LARYNX

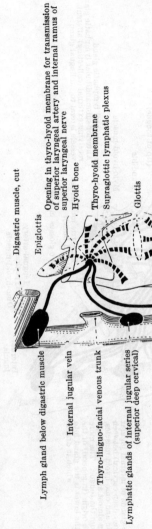

Digastric muscle, cut

Epiglottis

Opening in thyro-hyoid membrane for transmission
of superior laryngeal artery and internal ramus of
superior laryngeal nerve

Hyoid bone

Thyro-hyoid membrane

Supraglottic lymphatic plexus

Glottis

Infraglottic lymphatic plexus

Main lymph vessel passing through aperture in
crico-thyroid membrane

Prelaryngeal lymphatic gland

Lymphatic radicle passing laterally through the
crico-tracheal ligament

Isthmus of thyroid gland

Trachea

Pretracheal lymph gland

Lymph gland below digastric muscle

Internal jugular vein

Thyro-linguo-facial venous trunk

Lymphatic glands of internal jugular series
(superior deep cervical)

Thyroid cartilage

Recurrent laryngeal nerve

Lymphatic glands of internal jugular series
(superior deep cervical)

Lymphatic glands of recurrent chain, accompanying nerve

Afferent vessels going to lymphatic glands of internal
jugular chain (inferior deep cervical) and to
supraclavicular glands

PLATE 325.—LYMPHATICS OF THYROID GLAND

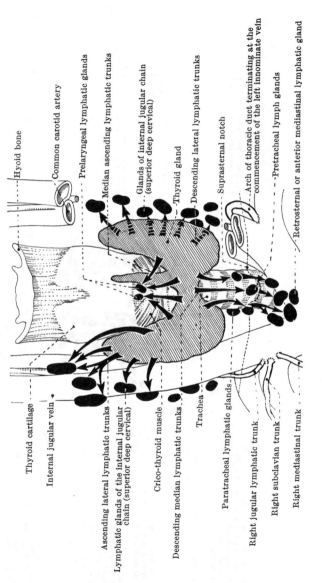

Hyoid bone

Common carotid artery

Prelaryngeal lymphatic glands

Median ascending lymphatic trunks

Glands of internal jugular chain (superior deep cervical)

Thyroid gland

Descending lateral lymphatic trunks

Suprasternal notch

Arch of thoracic duct terminating at the commencement of the left innominate vein

Pretracheal lymph glands

Retrosternal or anterior mediastinal lymphatic gland

Thyroid cartilage

Internal jugular vein

Ascending lateral lymphatic trunks

Lymphatic glands of the internal jugular chain (superior deep cervical)

Crico-thyroid muscle

Descending median lymphatic trunks

Trachea

Paratracheal lymphatic glands

Right jugular lymphatic trunk

Right subclavian trunk

Right mediastinal trunk

PLATE 326.—LYMPHATIC SYSTEM OF HEAD AND NECK

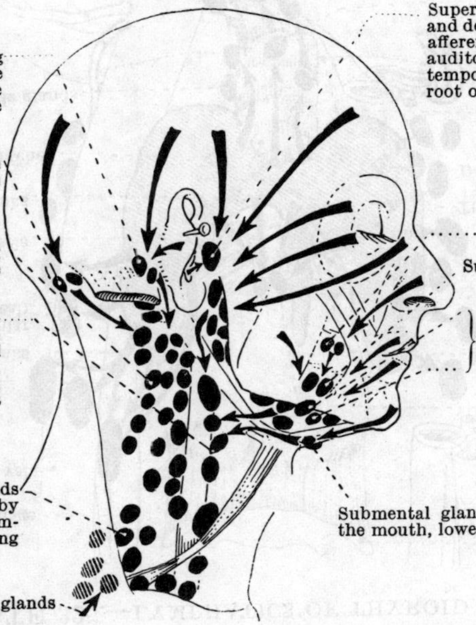

Superficial parotid [anterior auricular] lymph gland and deep parotid [parotid] glands receiving lymphatic afferent vessels from the tympanic cavity, external auditory meatus, lateral surface of auricle, superficial temporal and frontal lymphatics, and others from the root of the nose and from the eyelids

Buccinator group } superficial facial
Supramandibular group } lymph glands

Submandibular group receiving afferent vessels from the border of the anterior part of the tongue, gums, outer part of lower lip, upper lip, nose, and cheek

Submental glands receiving afferent vessels from the floor of the mouth, lower gums, middle of lower lip, and chin

Mastoid [posterior auricular] glands receiving afferent vessels from the posterior wall of the external auditory meatus, the medial surface of the auricle (the lobule excepted), and the temporal region

Occipital glands receiving lymph vessels from the occipital region

Posterior deep cervical chain receiving lymphatics from upper part and nape of neck and from intermediate glands

Anterior deep cervical chain receiving lymphatics from the thyroid gland, the nasal cavities, the larynx (in great part), the cervical portion of the trachea, the hard and soft palate, the middle and lower parts of the pharynx, the cervical part of the oesophagus, and almost all of the tongue

Inferior deep cervical (supraclavicular) glands receiving vessels from areas drained also by other cervical glands and some from the mammary region and lymph vessels accompanying the cephalic vein

Efferent vessels from axillary glands

PLATE 327.—LYMPH GLANDS OF AXILLA

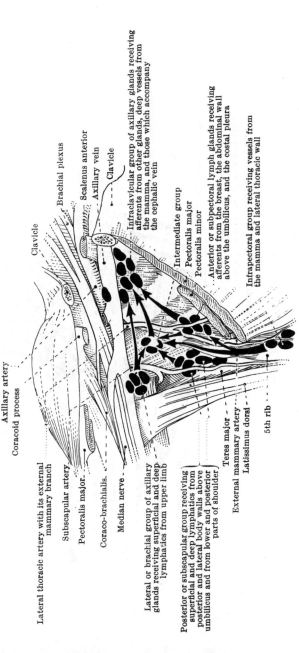

Axillary artery

Coracoid process

Clavicle

Brachial plexus

Scalenus anterior

Axillary vein

Clavicle

Infraclavicular group of axillary glands receiving
afferents from other glands, deep vessels from
the mamma, and those which accompany
the cephalic vein

Intermediate group

Pectoralis major

Pectoralis minor

Anterior or subpectoral lymph glands receiving
afferents from the breast, the abdominal wall
above the umbilicus, and the costal pleura

Infrapectoral group receiving vessels from
the mamma and lateral thoracic wall

5th rib

Latissimus dorsi

External mammary artery

Teres major

Median nerve

Coraco-brachialis.

Pectoralis major.

Subscapular artery

Lateral thoracic artery with its external
mammary branch

Lateral or brachial group of axillary
glands receiving superficial and deep
lymphatics from upper limb

Posterior or subscapular group receiving
superficial and deep lymphatics from
posterior and lateral body walls above
umbilicus and from lower and posterior
parts of shoulder

PLATE 328.—LYMPHATICS OF THE BREAST

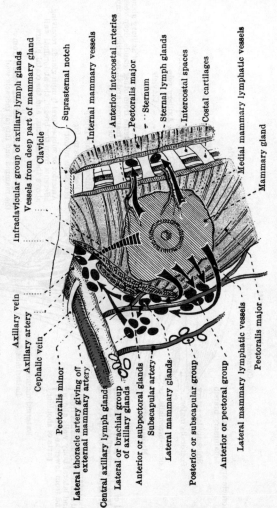

Axillary vein

Axillary artery

Cephalic vein

Pectoralis minor

Lateral thoracic artery giving off external mammary artery

Central axillary lymph glands

Lateral or brachial group of axillary glands

Anterior or subpectoral glands

Subscapular artery

Lateral mammary glands

Posterior or subscapular group

Anterior or pectoral group

Lateral mammary lymphatic vessels

Pectoralis major

Infraclavicular group of axillary lymph glands

Vessels from deep part of mammary gland

Clavicle

Suprasternal notch

Internal mammary vessels

Anterior intercostal arteries

Pectoralis major

Sternum

Sternal lymph glands

Intercostal spaces

Costal cartilages

Medial mammary lymphatic vessels

Mammary gland

Note.—The breast tissue is more extensive than shown

PLATE 329.—LYMPHATIC SYSTEM OF LUNGS

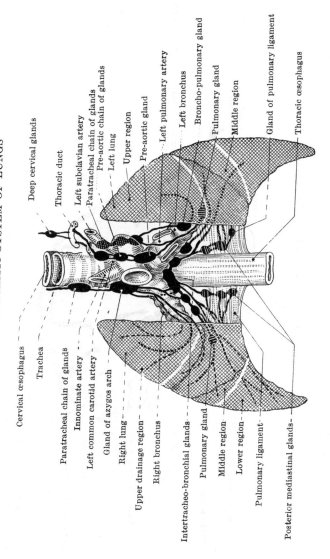

Cervical oesophagus

Deep cervical glands

Trachea

Thoracic duct

Paratracheal chain of glands

Left subclavian artery

Innominate artery

Paratracheal chain of glands

Left common carotid artery

Pre-aortic chain of glands

Gland of azygos arch

Left lung

Right lung

Upper region

Pre-aortic gland

Upper drainage region

Left pulmonary artery

Right bronchus

Left bronchus

Intertracheo-bronchial glands

Broncho-pulmonary gland

Pulmonary gland

Pulmonary gland

Middle region

Middle region

Lower region

Gland of pulmonary ligament

Pulmonary ligament

Thoracic oesophagus

Posterior mediastinal glands

PLATE 330.—LYMPHATICS OF STOMACH

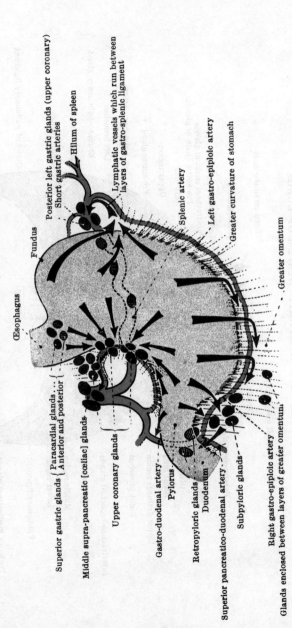

Œsophagus

Fundus

Posterior left gastric glands (upper coronary)

Short gastric arteries

Hilum of spleen

Lymphatic vessels which run between
layers of gastro-splenic ligament

Splenic artery

Left gastro-epiploic artery

Greater curvature of stomach

Greater omentum

Superior gastric glands { Paracardial glands...
                          Anterior and posterior

Middle supra-pancreatic [cœliac] glands·

Upper coronary glands

Gastro-duodenal artery

Retropyloric glands
Duodenum

Superior pancreatico-duodenal artery

Subpyloric glands

Right gastro-epiploic artery

Glands enclosed between layers of greater omentum

PLATE 331.—LYMPHATICS OF DUODENUM

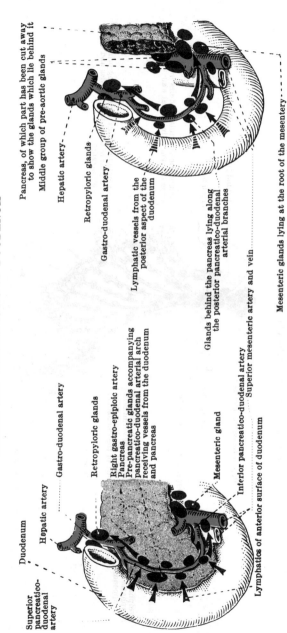

Pancreas, of which part has been cut away to show the glands which lie behind it

Middle group of pre-aortic glands

Hepatic artery

Retropyloric glands

Gastro-duodenal artery

Lymphatic vessels from the posterior aspect of the duodenum

Glands behind the pancreas lying along the posterior pancreatico-duodenal arterial branches

Mesenteric glands lying at the root of the mesentery

Superior pancreatico-duodenal artery

Duodenum

Hepatic artery

Gastro-duodenal artery

Retropyloric glands

Right gastro-epiploic artery
Pancreas
Pre-pancreatic glands accompanying pancreatico-duodenal arterial arch receiving vessels from the duodenum and pancreas

Mesenteric gland

Inferior pancreatico-duodenal artery
Superior mesenteric artery and vein

Lymphatics of anterior surface of duodenum

PLATE 332.—LYMPHATICS OF SMALL INTESTINE

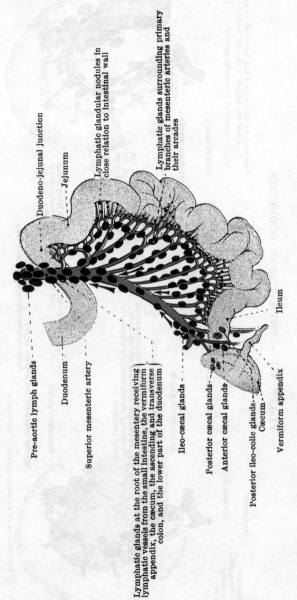

- Pre-aortic lymph glands
- Duodenum
- Superior mesenteric artery
- Duodeno-jejunal junction
- Jejunum
- Lymphatic glandular nodules in close relation to intestinal wall
- Lymphatic glands surrounding primary branches of mesenteric arteries and their arcades

Lymphatic glands at the root of the mesentery receiving lymphatic vessels from the small intestine, the vermiform appendix, the caecum, the ascending and transverse colon, and the lower part of the duodenum

- Ileo-caecal glands
- Posterior caecal glands
- Anterior caecal glands
- Posterior ileo-colic glands
- Caecum
- Vermiform appendix
- Ileum

PLATE 333.—LYMPHATICS OF LARGE INTESTINE

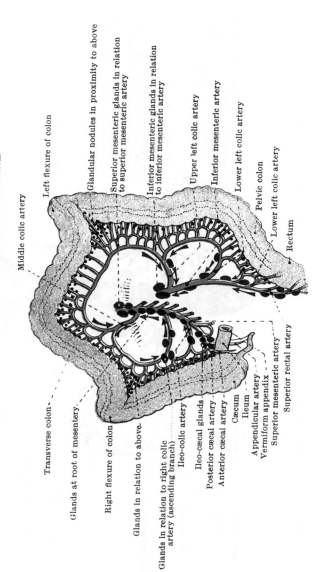

Middle colic artery

Left flexure of colon

Glandular nodules in proximity to above

Superior mesenteric glands in relation to superior mesenteric artery

Inferior mesenteric glands in relation to inferior mesenteric artery

Upper left colic artery

Inferior mesenteric artery

Lower left colic artery

Pelvic colon

Lower left colic artery

Rectum

Transverse colon

Glands at root of mesentery

Right flexure of colon

Glands in relation to above

Glands in relation to right colic artery (ascending branch)

Ileo-colic artery

Ileo-cæcal glands

Posterior cæcal artery

Anterior cæcal artery

Cæcum

Ileum

Appendicular artery

Vermiform appendix

Superior mesenteric artery

Superior rectal artery

PLATE 334.—LYMPHATICS OF THE KIDNEYS

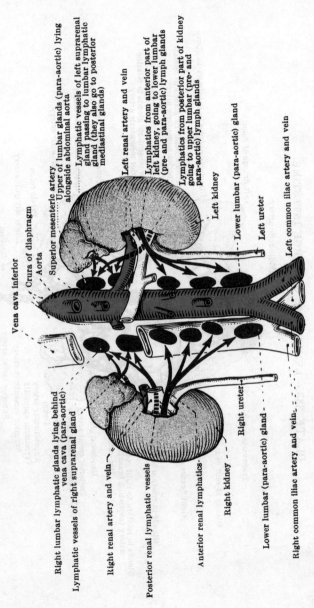

Vena cava inferior

Crura of diaphragm

Superior mesenteric artery

Aorta

Upper of lumbar glands (para-aortic) lying alongside abdominal aorta

Lymphatic vessels of left suprarenal gland passing to lumbar lymphatic gland (they also go to posterior mediastinal glands)

Left renal artery and vein

Lymphatics from anterior part of left kidney, going to lower lumbar (pre- and para-aortic) lymph glands

Lymphatics from posterior part of kidney going to upper lumbar (pre- and para-aortic) lymph glands

Left kidney

Lower lumbar (para-aortic) gland

Left ureter

Left common iliac artery and vein

Right lumbar lymphatic glands lying behind vena cava (para-aortic)

Lymphatic vessels of right suprarenal gland

Right renal artery and vein

Posterior renal lymphatic vessels

Anterior renal lymphatics

Right kidney

Right ureter

Lower lumbar (para-aortic) gland

Right common iliac artery and vein

PLATE 335.—AFFERENT LYMPHATIC VESSELS OF UPPER PRE-AORTIC GLANDS

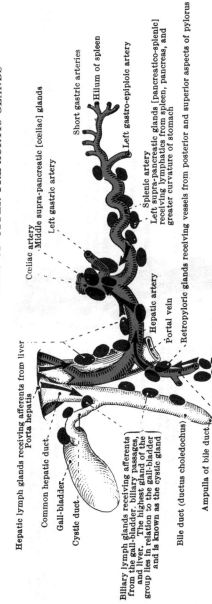

Hepatic lymph glands receiving afferents from liver
Porta hepatis

Common hepatic duct.

Gall-bladder.

Cystic duct.

Biliary lymph glands receiving afferents from the gall-bladder, biliary passages, and liver. The highest gland of the group lies in relation to the gall-bladder and is known as the cystic gland

Bile duct (ductus choledochus)

Ampulla of bile duct

Right gastro-epiploic artery

Cœliac artery
Middle supra-pancreatic [cœliac] glands

Left gastric artery

Short gastric arteries

Hilum of spleen

Left gastro-epiploic artery

Splenic artery
Left supra-pancreatic glands [pancreatico-splenic] receiving lymphatics from spleen, pancreas, and greater curvature of stomach

Hepatic artery

Portal vein

Retropyloric glands receiving vessels from posterior and superior aspects of pylorus

Subpyloric glands receiving vessels from inferior part of stomach and upper part of greater omentum

PLATE 336.—PRE-AORTIC LYMPH GLANDS

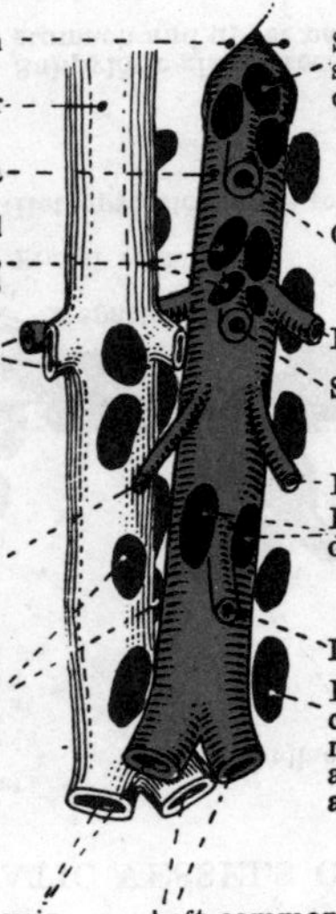

Crura of the diaphragm

Vena cava inferior

Aorta

Middle group, receiving lymphatics from the small intestine, appendix and cæcum, ascending colon, transverse colon, and some from the pancreas

Right renal artery and vein {

Right testicular artery

Right para-aortic glands—pre- and retro-venous, receiving lymphatics from the same parts as the left chain; those of the right genital organs passing chiefly to the pre-venous glands, those from the pelvic wall chiefly to the retro-venous chain

Right common iliac artery and vein

Superior group, receiving lymphatics from liver, stomach, spleen, pancreas, first part of duodenum, gall-bladder, cystic duct, hepatic duct, part of bile duct, and pylorus

Cœliac artery

Left renal artery

Superior mesenteric artery

Left testicular artery

Inferior group, receiving lymphatics from the descending and pelvic colon and the rectum

Inferior mesenteric artery

Left para-aortic glands, receiving lymphatics from the left common iliac groups, the left testicle, epididymis, etc. (in the male), the left half of the uterus (in the female), the left kidney and suprarenal body [gland], and muscles of the posterior abdominal wall

Left common iliac artery and vein

PLATE 337.—LYMPHATICS OF UTERUS

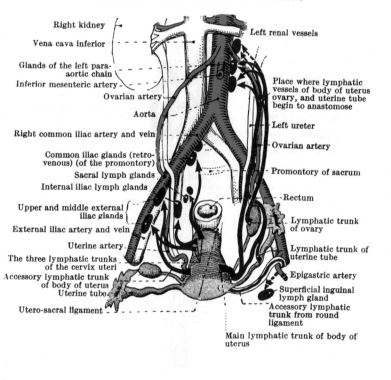

Right kidney

Vena cava inferior

Glands of the left para-aortic chain

Inferior mesenteric artery

Ovarian artery

Aorta

Right common iliac artery and vein

Common iliac glands (retro-venous) (of the promontory)

Sacral lymph glands

Internal iliac lymph glands

Upper and middle external iliac glands

External iliac artery and vein

Uterine artery

The three lymphatic trunks of the cervix uteri

Accessory lymphatic trunk of body of uterus

Uterine tube

Utero-sacral ligament

Left renal vessels

Place where lymphatic vessels of body of uterus ovary, and uterine tube begin to anastomose

Left ureter

Ovarian artery

Promontory of sacrum

Rectum

Lymphatic trunk of ovary

Lymphatic trunk of uterine tube

Epigastric artery

Superficial inguinal lymph gland

Accessory lymphatic trunk from round ligament

Main lymphatic trunk of body of uterus

PLATE 338.—THORACIC DUCT AND ITS TRIBUTARIES

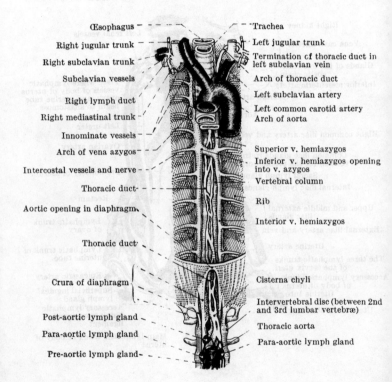

Œsophagus

Right jugular trunk

Right subclavian trunk

Subclavian vessels

Right lymph duct

Right mediastinal trunk

Innominate vessels

Arch of vena azygos

Intercostal vessels and nerve

Thoracic duct

Aortic opening in diaphragm

Thoracic duct

Crura of diaphragm

Post-aortic lymph gland

Para-aortic lymph gland

Pre-aortic lymph gland

Trachea

Left jugular trunk

Termination of thoracic duct in left subclavian vein

Arch of thoracic duct

Left subclavian artery

Left common carotid artery
Arch of aorta

Superior v. hemiazygos

Inferior v. hemiazygos opening into v. azygos

Vertebral column

Rib

Interior v. hemiazygos

Cisterna chyli

Intervertebral disc (between 2nd and 3rd lumbar vertebræ)

Thoracic aorta

Para-aortic lymph gland

PLATE 339.—CONTENTS OF MEDIASTINUM—SEEN FROM BEHIND

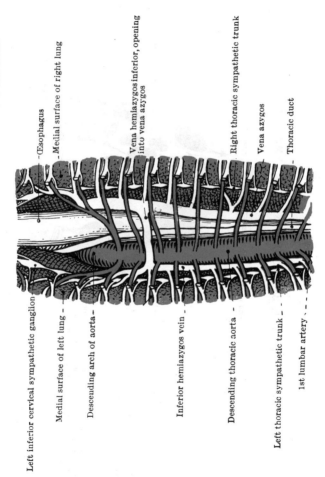

Œsophagus

Medial surface of right lung

Vena hemiazygos inferior, opening into vena azygos

Right thoracic sympathetic trunk

Vena azygos

Thoracic duct

Left inferior cervical sympathetic ganglion

Medial surface of left lung

Descending arch of aorta

Inferior hemiazygos vein

Descending thoracic aorta

Left thoracic sympathetic trunk

1st lumbar artery

PLATE 340.—COMMON ILIAC LYMPH GLANDS

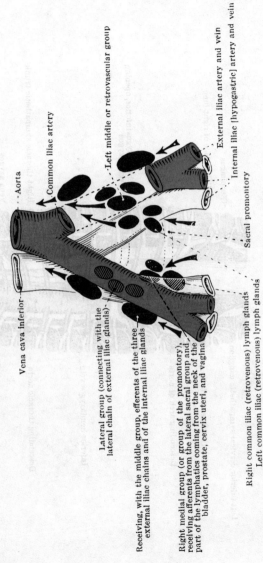

Vena cava inferior

Aorta

Common iliac artery

Left middle or retrovascular group

External iliac artery and vein

Internal iliac [hypogastric] artery and vein

Sacral promontory

Lateral group (connecting with the lateral chain of external iliac glands)

Receiving, with the middle group, efferents of the three external iliac chains and of the internal iliac glands

Right medial group (or group of the promontory), receiving afferents from the lateral sacral group and part of the lymphatics coming from the neck of the bladder, prostate, cervix uteri, and vagina

Right common iliac (retrovenous) lymph glands
Left common iliac (retrovenous) lymph glands

PLATE 341.—SUPERFICIAL INGUINAL GLANDS

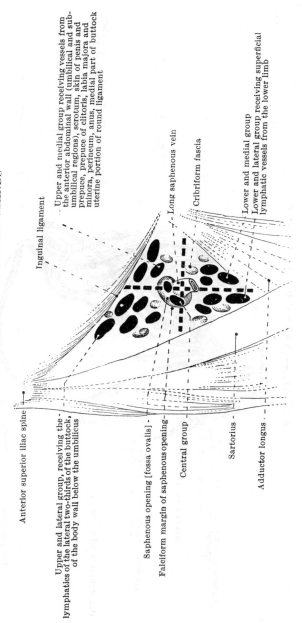

Anterior superior iliac spine

Upper and lateral group, receiving the lymphatics of the lateral two-thirds of the buttock, of the body wall below the umbilicus

Saphenous opening [fossa ovalis]

Falciform margin of saphenous opening

Central group

Sartorius

Adductor longus

Inguinal ligament

Upper and medial group receiving vessels from the anterior abdominal wall (umbilical and sub-prepuce, prepuce of penis, skin of penis and minora, perineum, anus, medial part of buttock uterine portion of round ligament

Long saphenous vein

Cribriform fascia

Lower and medial group

Lower and lateral group receiving superficial lymphatic vessels from the lower limb

PLATE 342.—LYMPHATICS OF RECTUM

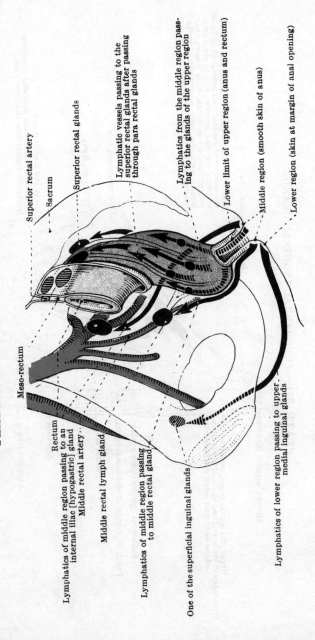

Meso-rectum

Rectum

Lymphatics of middle region passing to an internal iliac [hypogastric] gland

Middle rectal artery

Middle rectal lymph gland

Lymphatics of middle region passing to middle rectal gland

One of the superficial inguinal glands

Lymphatics of lower region passing to upper medial inguinal glands

Superior rectal artery

Sacrum

Superior rectal glands

Lymphatic vessels passing to the superior rectal glands after passing through para rectal glands

Lymphatics from the middle region passing to the glands of the upper region

Lower limit of upper region (anus and rectum)

Middle region (smooth skin of anus)

Lower region (skin at margin of anal opening)

PLATE 343.—EXTERNAL AND INTERNAL ILIAC [HYPOGASTRIC] LYMPHATIC GLANDS

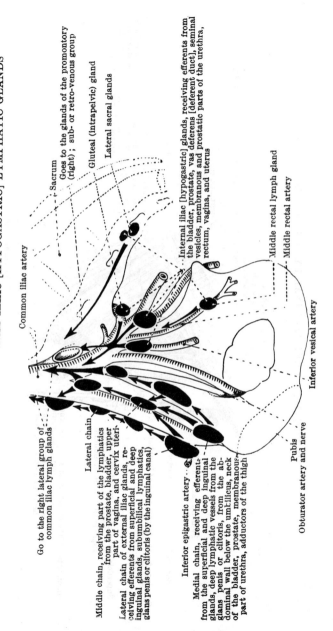

Go to the right lateral group of
common iliac lymph glands

Common iliac artery

Sacrum

Goes to the glands of the promontory
(right) ; sub- or retro-venous group

Gluteal (intrapelvic) gland

Lateral sacral glands

Internal iliac [hypogastric] glands, receiving efferents from
the bladder, prostate, vas deferens [deferent duct], seminal
vesicles, membranous and prostatic parts of the urethra,
rectum, vagina, and uterus

Middle chain, receiving part of the lymphatics
from the prostate, bladder, upper
part of vagina, and cervix uteri

Lateral chain

Lateral chain of external iliac glands, receiving efferents from superficial and deep
inguinal glands, subumbilical lymphatics,
glans penis or clitoris (by the inguinal canal)

Inferior epigastric artery

Medial chain, receiving efferents
from the superficial and deep inguinal
glands, deep lymphatic vessels from the
glans penis or clitoris, from the abdominal wall below the umbilicus, neck
of the bladder, prostate, membranous
part of urethra, adductors of the thigh

Obturator artery and nerve

Pubis

Inferior vesical artery

Middle rectal lymph gland

Middle rectal artery

PLATE 344.—DEEP INGUINAL LYMPH GLANDS

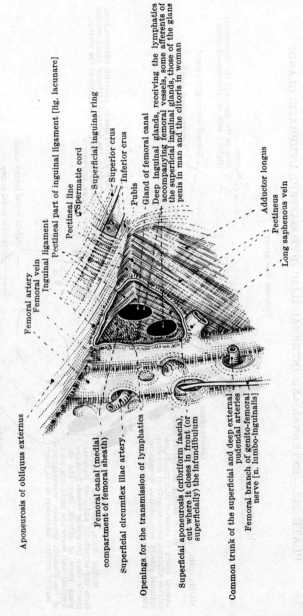

Aponeurosis of obliquus externus

Pectineal part of inguinal ligament [lig. lacunare]

Pectineal line

Spermatic cord

Superior crus

Inferior crus

Pubis

Gland of femoral canal

Deep inguinal glands, receiving the lymphatics accompanying femoral vessels, some afferents of the superficial inguinal glands, those of the glans penis in man and the clitoris in woman

Femoral artery
Femoral vein
Inguinal ligament

Superficial inguinal ring

Adductor longus

Pectineus

Long saphenous vein

Femoral canal (medial compartment of femoral sheath)

Superficial circumflex iliac artery

Openings for the transmission of lymphatics

Superficial aponeurosis (cribriform fascia), cut where it closes in front (or superficially) the infundibulum

Common trunk of the superficial and deep external pudendal arteries

Femoral branch of genito-femoral nerve [n. lumbo-inguinalis]

PLATE 345.—POPLITEAL GLANDS

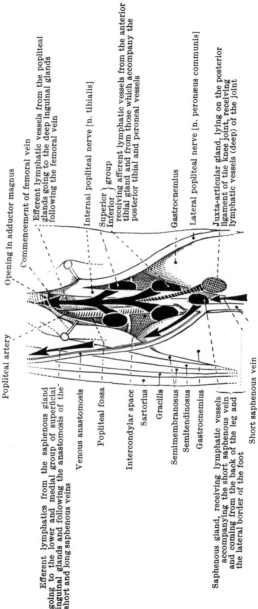

Popliteal artery

Opening in adductor magnus

Commencement of femoral vein

Efferent lymphatic vessels from the popliteal
glands going to the deep inguinal glands
following the femoral vein

Internal popliteal nerve [n. tibialis]

Superior } group
Inferior
receiving afferent lymphatic vessels from the anterior
tibial gland and from those which accompany the
posterior tibial and peroneal vessels

Gastrocnemius

Lateral popliteal nerve [n. peronæus communis]

Juxta-articular gland, lying on the posterior
ligament of the knee joint, receiving
lymphatic vessels (deep) of the joint

Efferent lymphatics from the saphenous gland
going to the lower and medial group of superficial
inguinal glands and following the anastomosis of the
short and long saphenous veins

Venous anastomosis

Popliteal fossa

Intercondylar space

Sartorius

Gracilis

Semimembranosus

Semitendinosus

Gastrocnemius

Saphenous gland, receiving lymphatic vessels
accompanying the short saphenous vein
and coming from the back of the leg and
the lateral border of the foot

Short saphenous vein

INDEX

347